D1396866

We Walk the World

World

A Journey of Healing

By Lewis G. Zirkle, MD

ISBN-10: 1976239214
ISBN-13: 978-1976239212

Dedication

To the SIGN Family

Contents

Acknowledgments

Sara, my wife, has been a quiet source of strength and tolerance through 54 years of our marriage. Our three daughters Elizabeth, Molly, and Julie are very supportive of SIGN and our goals. Sara and our daughters have all contributed to the advancement of SIGN in different ways. Our daughters and nine grandchildren have all placed SIGN Nails in sawbones, including placement of the distal interlocking screws. My father, whose picture hangs in the SIGN Manufacturing Area, and my mother gave me needed advice in the early days of SIGN. Dad shared his engineering experience during our daily phone calls when he was still living.

Randy Huebner and his wife Mary have been supporters of SIGN, providing knowledge and needed advice. Both of them continue to help SIGN in many ways.

Jeanne Dillner has provided organization and implementation to build the SIGN Staff into a highly functioning team. Her excellence in performance and commitment to SIGN was recently recognized by the SIGN Board. The SIGN Staff are enthusiastic about their jobs and very proficient. Each member is a pleasure to work with.

The SIGN Board Members have all contributed in different ways to the success of SIGN.

SIGN Surgeons throughout the world have contributed to the success of the 200,000 SIGN Surgeries. They are innovative and give of their time and skills to care for the poor. I emphasized their many innovations in the book.

Dr. Clay Wertheimer made excellent revisions to my poorly written story. He spent many hours editing, and I am grateful for this time spent. Burney Garelick provided editorial advice.

Members of our dedicated SIGN Staff are very enthusiastic and capable. We all work together toward our goal. Ryan Smith edited the book using many parameters and Sherry Nelson provided valuable assistance in layout and illustrations.

SIGN has many faithful committed donors including Kiwanis, The Wyss Foundation, generous private foundations, and many individual donors.

Diversity trumps ability, according to Scott Page, and the SIGN Journey is propelled by a diverse group of people with a common goal of providing equality of fracture care throughout the world.

Foreword

"Commitment is an act, not a word."
—Jean-Paul Sartre

Thank you for choosing to read about the journey one man took to correct a disabling inequality. Writing this book has been a long, arduous task, but those of us who work closely with Dr. Zirkle are thankful to him for taking the time to put into words the genesis of this amazing journey and to convey his passions and philosophies, which have resulted in hundreds of thousands of healed limbs.

What makes a person like Dr. Zirkle desire to solve a problem on such a large scale? Was Dr. Zirkle predisposed to commit his inheritance and surgical expertise to heal the poorest humans of the world? Or was it the series of experiences of watching his father cross racial barriers, or Dr. Baker taking him to serve the poor in the deep south, or the little boy in Vietnam whose father gave the gift of a mango?

All these attributes and experiences led him to the ultimate impetus for SIGN, which he calls 'the man in the bed.' Discovering this poor man's experience of laying for three years in traction was the aha for Dr. Zirkle. At that moment, it was clear to him that implants needed to be included with the education in order for patients to heal. But the implants needed hadn't been designed yet. The challenge to provide a sustainable supply of relevant implants was daunting. Another man might have quit right there. But Dr. Zirkle chose to remain true to his commitment and, with stubborn persistence fueled by the passion of finding a solution for patients like the man in the bed, he widened the path of his journey to find a sustainable solution for healing the poor.

His natural scientific curiosity and confidence birthed the idea that he could design the devices and manufacture them in his home town. He chose to hire people who were mission minded and who had no orthopaedic design experience, so that we could all start with fresh ideas. All of us were inspired and naively optimistic that we could succeed in helping Dr. Zirkle develop these devices—and by golly we did. None of us were burdened by the bureaucracy of the larger implant companies. Our focus was on designing and manufacturing the devices as quickly as possible. The urgency was real and invigorating. Every nail we made and shipped meant a patient was going to walk again.

Dr. Zirkle's designs always incorporated the ideas of the overseas doctors. As the local experts and users, their input was required to ensure that the implants and instruments were designed specifically for the low-resourced hospitals they work in. This inclusive mindset built trust and better products for their patients. Thousands of grateful surgeons attribute the growth of orthopaedics in their country to Dr. Zirkle's generosity with implants, knowledge, and faithful mentorship.

"It's ok to live a life that others don't understand" —anonymous

Dr. Zirkle's faith in the quality of surgery that would be performed overcame the early naysayers who insisted that the overseas doctors would not have the intellect or skill to perform internal fixation. In the thousands of surgeries and hundreds of hospital operating rooms

I've been in over the years, I've witnessed that the SIGN Surgeons and nurses are compassionate, dedicated, and employ sound surgical techniques. Dr. Zirkle's review of the surgical database confirms the creative and successful surgical prowess of these men and women.

Inevitably, there are times when Dr. Zirkle's burden for the poor creates a tension in his relationships with family, friends, colleagues, and SIGN Surgeons and Staff. Not many people understand his work ethic and frequently recommend that he take a break and relax.

How can he relax when there are more accidents occurring every day? What about the patients suffering in Iraq? Or the Afghan surgeons who need us to deploy more SIGN Sets in the war-torn areas of their nation? Or surgeons in South Sudan who are operating without electricity in their hospital? In his mind, the patients in the bed need these new devices and now! To his credit, he can't let go of the empathy he feels for the patients who fear that their limb may never heal.

Dr. Zirkle's ability to perform with excellence in surgery, develop meaningful educational programs, and create relevant and innovative devices offsets any tensions generated by the sense of urgency he feels for these suffering souls.

Like the surgeons overseas, I've grown as a person and as a leader from walking this journey with Dr. Zirkle. The list is long, but here are some of my favorite lessons: how to handle 'many balls in the air' without becoming frozen with stress, that it is good to set and reset priorities as you get new information, and always strive to have the right balance of compassion and efficiency (heavier on the compassion).

This journey has led me away from vacations and catching the latest sitcom to joyful experiences like seeing my international friends succeed at a new surgical skill. A special memory was witnessing one SIGN friend stand with pride next to Dr. Zirkle while we each received a medal of honor from the president of Afghanistan.

I've been privileged to watch a parent's face relax with relief when they see the x-ray that shows their child's femur is held securely in place and starting to heal. No sitcom compares to watching a son look lovingly at his elderly mother who is finally able to walk again because her hip is repaired—all with the implants made just a few hundred feet from my office back home. These memories are worth so much more than those derived from any leisurely vacation.

Serving with Dr. Zirkle at the helm these last 18 years has been continuously life improving for me, our staff, our board and supporters, the SIGN Surgeons, and tens of thousands of families across the globe. I look forward to remaining on this journey with him for many years to come. Enjoy *your* reading journey!

Jeanne Dillner

CEO of SIGN Fracture Care International

* * * * *

The following notes from SIGN Surgeons, express how they have been educated, equipped, and inspired by Dr. Zirkle.

When I was an orthopaedics resident of Yangon General Hospital in 1994, I met Dr. Lewis Zirkle, who visited to our hospital. We made cases discussion with him, and we had opportunity to learn from him about knowledge of orthopaedics related with presented cases. We heard that he was a military doctor and served as a battlefield medical officer in the Vietnam War, and that he wanted to change the plight of poor patients with broken bones. He established the SIGN and started to help to the poor patients around the world, including Myanmar.

In 2002 Dr. Zirkle came to visit our hospital, and he operated a femoral fracture patient in the emergency operation theater. He taught our team how to operate with SIGN Nail on fracture patients. From that time, Yangon General Hospital started to use SIGN Implants for long bone fracture patients. Since then, SIGN continuously supplies and donates the implants for our poor patients. There are nearly to 4,000 patients in our hospital who were operated with using SIGN Nails for their fractures.

Apart from donating the nails, which are aimed for long bone fractures, SIGN donates other instruments (plates, screws, external fixators, pelvis operating sets, some kinds of medications). All these are very helpful and make benefit to our people most of them are not affordable to costly implants and drugs.

When we started the SIGN Program in our hospital, we sent the patient data into webpage of SIGN and faculties of SIGN responded to us with email about the result of patients operated with SIGN Implants. We have contact to them with email and they give suggestions, constructive discussion, and share their updated knowledge to group of surgeons who are primarily performing operations. We have our hospital SIGN Surgical Database in which more than 3,000 patients' facts and figures are recorded.

SIGN contributes to us the activities of continuous professional development by inviting Myanmar orthopaedic surgeons to the annual SIGN Conference held in Richland, USA. We have opportunity to meet and make friends with international surgeons attending the conference. These surgeons share their experience and knowledge in different ways (presentations, workshops, poster shows, and free talks). During the conference, SIGN donates implants, medical literature, and other surgical things to the group of surgeons. The literature and surgical textbooks donated by SIGN are very effective to improve our knowledge. We have limited facilities to get highly prized surgical textbooks.

SIGN members, including Dr. Zirkle, regularly visit our hospital and contribute educational development, care of patients, and bring SIGN Implants with their baggage. We use these surgical apparatuses for not only Myanmar people but also to patient from China.

SIGN has no boundaries. Now, SIGN Programs are in nine hospitals of Myanmar including two military hospitals. SIGN has no barriers and no discrimination for fracture care. Equality of fracture care round the world is a reality for us. SIGN saves thousands of limbs and many lives of Myanmar people. The SIGN Program brings our patients, from unaffordable to affordable, from disabled to mobile, from cry to smile, and from desperate to prosperous.

Dr. Aung Thein Htay
Yangon, Myanmar

＊ ＊ ＊ ＊ ＊

Before I met Dr. Zirkle, orthopaedic surgery used to take a day of preparation with templating before finally venturing into the very bloody procedure of inserting the nail. We did not have a full-time orthopaedic surgeon, so the two of us general surgery residents gained whatever orthopaedic skill during the visit of short-term visitors. The manual was clear enough but we took forever to understand the details. I remember once, I had placed a retrograde SIGN Nail with a posterior convexity instead of anterior, and Dr. Zirkle commented that it was to be the reverse. That has stuck in my mind till now; how he looks at every single case of the database to every detail. His commitment and devotion to detail about each patient reminds me as I manage each patient. As a surgeon, I feel humbled that patients entrust their lives to our competence, and as such we must treat them with equal devotion and commitment. This comment from the post-op x-ray on the database was over 12 years ago and has stayed with me ever since. I have also learnt discipline. I have seen programs shut down because they do not report cases or follow-ups on the database as expected. As surgeons, we have to be disciplined as a mark of seriousness.

Despite this malorientation in the case I mention above, the fracture still healed very well. The SIGN Nail has over the years become "a nail without a specific indication." To me it depends on the skill and creativity of the surgeon to make it work in less indicated situations. Surprisingly the SIGN Engineers receive such attempts with excitement and interest rather than questioning or indignation. The SIGN Surgeons are made to be part of the owners of the system; their contribution is valued and considered. I have had no need for an alternative fracture fixation system of treating long bone fractures than the SIGN Nail. More so, the nails are always available at no cost, so no patient fails to receive a fracture fixation simply because of lack of funds. In many situations we successfully treat almost all tibia fractures closed without a C-arm, as well as even some femur fractures. The nail design has probably surpassed its originally intended indications, and the SIGN Engineers keep improving on it every day. I believe in a few years the SIGN Nail will be the dominant implant in low and middle income countries (where healthcare is not profit driven by insurance companies).

SIGN Surgeons are exposed to world-class conference courses and workshops, which would be difficult to access by individual effort. We also have the opportunity to present papers of local experiences to an international audience. The SIGN Conference is the only conference in the world with a beautiful mix of advances in surgery and current realities in the developing world. As once mentioned, the SIGN Conference is a "United Nations," the most diverse group involved in a unique practice with similar intentions of meeting the needs of both the affluent and the most vulnerable people with standard trauma care. This no doubt aligns with the vision of SIGN—equality of fracture care throughout the world.

Dr. Henry Ndasi
Mutengene, Cameroon

★ ★ ★ ★ ★

In late 2009, I was a medical student in Peshawar, Pakistan. I wanted to learn and share. I was interested in doing research in orthopaedics but I lacked direction. My '5-Year Plan' back then was to be able to present my research at an international conference or get a publication in an internationally acclaimed orthopaedic journal. Since the US has always been one of the leading countries for research; I made my '5-Year Plan' tougher by presenting in a conference in the US and being published in the US. The only problem was that I lacked public speaking skills and I was very shy. The very thought of standing and speaking in front of people would send a shiver down my spine.

Fast forward to September, 2010 in Richland, WA. I met Dr. Lewis G. Zirkle and he encouraged me to present my research at the Annual SIGN Conference. I was just an introverted young medical student attending my first orthopaedic conference. I didn't know how to hide my fears, nor did I know that this audience will be my strength. I was nervous throughout my talk but I was inspired by Dr. Zirkle's demeanor.

I never expected this to be a life-changing experience. A month later, I was in Baltimore, MD, at the Orthopaedic Trauma Association conference. I was quizzed by two of the leading orthopaedic surgeons in North America regarding my research. I thought I did okay with their questions, but then I saw my father and Dr. Zirkle, who both had beaming smiles. Their handshakes meant that the shy medical student is now an eloquent presenter.

Since 2010, I have presented 17 research papers in various international conferences and published five research articles in orthopaedic journals. In between all this, I became the first Pakistani resident to present a research paper at American Academy of Orthopaedic Surgeons annual meeting and have the highest number of presentations at SIGN Conference since 2010.

The applause I receive whenever I finish off each of my presentations are actually for people who encouraged me to soar to the heights, which I had never imagined before. That applause is all for my mentor, Dr. Lewis Zirkle.

Dr. Faseeh Shahab
Peshwar, Pakistan

* * * * *

We are so thankful to SIGN Fracture Care International for its dedication and willingness to support orthopaedic and trauma programs in third world countries.

Before the advent of a SIGN Program in my hospital, we had very few options on how to treat long bone fractures and other complex fractures related to long bone fractures, including open fractures.

This situation led to more morbidity, much higher costs to the families, and less productivity as patients had to stay in the hospital for long time to get some healing before being discharged. These patients were not necessarily healed and did not get back into the normal function of their limbs because of the nature of the injury that could not be treated by cast, traction, or other treatment.

In 2013, we saw miracles when Lew Zirkle, the Founder and President of SIGN and Jeanne Dillner CEO of SIGN visited us for the first time.

Patients who had unattended fractures for more than five years, complex fractures that we used to apply traction were operated by Dr. Zirkle. Knowing that Dr. Zirkle will visit us, we had to ask him if could invite residents from nearby teaching hospital, for him it is always a pleasure to share knowledge with young and other ortho-paedic surgeons.

So we had an opportunity to operate and learn different SIGN Techniques from Dr. Zirkle. Now cases that we used to think were impossible to be fixed, are no longer a problem in our center.

Through SIGN many patients get treated well, with less mor-bidity, shorter hospital stays, and less costs to the family. They have better quality of lives if treated by SIGN Implants. SIGN Implants have revolutionized our thinking in terms of fracture care.

Thank you Dr. Zirkle, Jeanne, all SIGN Staff, and all SIGN Surgeons all over the world.

Dr. Sam Kiwesa
Moshi, Tanzania

* * * * *

Afghanistan is a mountainous country located in the heart of Asia whose people are suffering from poverty and war for more than three decades. Besides lacking other structural basics, the health sector is severely damaged. With increased numbers of gunshot fractures, road traffic accidents, and natural disasters like earthquake, floods, and landslides there was little opportunity for these patients to be treated correctly.

Before Dr. Zirkle came to visit our country, we had few centers and small number of orthopaedic surgeons in Afghanistan. The lack of training and instruments and implants was a big challenge for us. During the Russian invasion, they introduced Ilizarov's external fixation technique, but it was only available for a few centers, primarily in the Army.

In 2007, Dr. Zirkle made his first visit to Afghanistan to establish SIGN Programs in Kabul at the major civilian and military hospitals. He personally trained the surgeons working in Kabul to perform the SIGN Technique.

He returned in 2008 to attend the first Afghan SIGN Conference held in Kabul. For the first time in the history of Afghanistan, we gathered hundreds of orthopaedic surgeons from all over the country and established Afghan Orthopaedic Association. Dr. Zirkle trained these surgeons directly in sawbones workshops and live surgeries. With the support of Dr. Zirkle and SIGN we have started more programs in many other provinces. My team has traveled and performed surgeries with each new program in Afghanistan.

In 2015, Dr. Zirkle returned for the second Afghan SIGN Conference in Kabul which was more successful and many more surgeons were trained personally by Dr. Zirkle.

The president of Afghanistan, Dr. Ashraf Ghani, awarded the highest Medal of Honor of Afghanistan, the Allama Sayed Jamaluddin Afghan Medal, to Dr. Zirkle and me for the service of poor in our country.

Now Afghanistan has the most SIGN Programs in the world with more than 20 active programs that treated almost 8,000 fractures during last ten years.

Our practices have less need for Ilizarov for treating deformity as we do the lengthening on SIGN Nails, and under supervision of Dr. Zirkle we have suggested many new methods and innovations of the SIGN System. We shortened the time of surgery for long bones to few minutes, which shows the expertise of Afghan surgeons. We have abandoned the use of plates on long bones and decreased the complications to less than 2 percent.

On behalf of the people of Afghanistan, especially orthopaedic surgeons, we are all thankful for the unlimited efforts of Dr. Lew Zirkle, who is helping us to treat the poor in Afghanistan. May God bless him and his team with a long life and more success in his life to serve the poor around the world.

Dr. Ismail Wardak
Kabul, Afghanistan

* * * * *

SIGN has provided us with the best tool (SIGN Nail), taught us to perform surgeries the right way (EDUCATION), and encouraged us to study ways on how to make things better (RESEARCH). All over the world SIGN has touched peoples' lives, changed families, and united orthopaedic surgeons from different races and cultures to create a priceless and invaluable virtue—hope for humanity.

Dr. Jun Valera
Davao City, Philippines

Preface

The Journey of
SIGN Fracture Care International

The journey of SIGN has taken many twists and turns, even some backward steps, as we have pursued our vision of creating equality of fracture care throughout the world. Our model of education plus donation of appropriate implants was developed after recognizing my mistake in not validating early efforts to help the injured poor in Indonesia. We now validate our results by evaluating reports including x-rays of the majority of SIGN Surgeries. The database facilitates evaluation of results and reveals innovative ideas from surgeons around the world. We are continually improving the database to make it more accessible in areas of decreased Internet reception. Recent changes devised by our skilled SIGN Staff will facilitate communication between SIGN Surgeons around the world.

The journey of SIGN can be compared to a swarm of fish, birds, or bats. These swarms move as a unit through group thinking rather than individual decisions. SIGN is not a hierarchy and we consider all suggestions from SIGN Surgeons, SIGN Staff, and engineers throughout the world. The needs of injured poor patients always guide the direction and speed of the SIGN Swarm. Luck, persistence, diversity, and determination all play a role in the SIGN Journey. New ideas to increase the quality of care for the injured poor can be compared to a bubble. This bubble expands as others add ideas until these innovations mature and the aha moment occurs—often simultaneously in different parts of the world.

The epidemic of trauma, especially road traffic accidents, continues to increase. Inexpensive motorcycles have accelerated the number and severity of the injuries. The injured poor have no choice in their treatment. Therefore, the SIGN Family must provide the best care available. Over 5,000 surgeons throughout the world treat the poor in more than 50 countries. These surgeons have used SIGN Education and Implants to heal more than 200,000 patients. I feel privileged to participate in their journey and to tell the story of SIGN Fracture Care International.

Chapter 1

A Mango

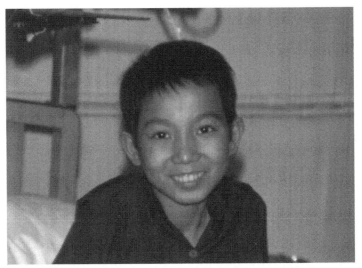

Nguyen had a dislocated knee, many burns, and a radiant smile, despite painful treatment to straighten his leg.

In 1968, Nguyen, a 10-year-old boy, was transported by Medevac helicopter to the 93rd Evacuation Hospital in Vietnam. He had been burned by napalm. His knee was scarred and stuck at a 90-degree angle. He could not walk and had pain when he moved his leg. I admitted him to the Vietnamese ward of the hospital, where I placed him in traction by placing pins through the bones on both sides of the knee. We gradually increased the weight on these pins to gradually increase his knee motion. He needed to be able to straighten the joint in order to walk and live a normal life.

We increased the traction force based on how much pain the boy could stand. This required teamwork between Nguyen and me, and we came to know each other quite well. We knew we had to consider the long-term advantages of increasing his knee motion versus the short-term pain he would have to endure. Nguyen was very brave. He usually had a smile on his face, except when the weight was increased. But he never complained.

When his knee reached full motion and he could walk again, it was time for him to go home. A Vietnamese woman on the same ward notified his family. His father came to the hospital by bus. It was an emotional reunion for father and son. When Nguyen's father arrived, he carried a mango. Then, with tears in his eyes, he offered the fruit to me. As I accepted it, I saw a deep thumb print and realized how tightly he had grasped the mango during his bus ride. When I looked up, Nguyen's father was walking into the sunset, his arm around his son.

I, too, had many emotions as I watched father and son walk into the waning daylight toward the bus stop. Nguyen and I had become friends because we had a common goal of straightening his leg. We didn't know each other's language, so we couldn't communicate verbally. We were able to understand each other by facial expressions, gestures, and compassion. We knew that we were working toward a common goal, and we got there. I never saw the boy again, but he had a great influence on me. The satisfaction of caring for a fellow human being who had no other means of treatment has motivated me to help patients all over the world.

While treating injuries of both US military personnel and Vietnamese civilians, I became more and more distressed. It was apparent that the injured on both sides would suffer long-term disability. Even now, more than 40 years later, some US veterans of the Vietnam War still exhibit Post Traumatic Stress Disorder (PTSD) that ruins their lives. I am sure the Vietnamese wounded also have many residual effects, both physical and mental. My emotional reaction to the war was emerging rage, but I had no time to vent and no one to vent to. Anger provides a positive emotional release, but it can become a negative force in our lives. Anger must be channeled to fix the problem before it becomes destructive.

People in all countries continue to be victims of circumstances over which they have no control. The World Health Organization reports that "injuries are a neglected epidemic in developing countries, causing more than five million deaths each year, roughly equal to the number of deaths from HIV/AIDS, malaria and tuberculosis combined."[1] Road traffic accidents and trauma are especially prevalent in places where people do not have access to proper treatment. My experience with Nguyen taught me that people are not statistics or metrics—but human beings like you and me. They have dreams that too often are shattered in the blink of an eye or by the break of a bone. They dream their children will go to school, get good jobs, and lift the family out of poverty. They dream they can walk and sleep through the night without pain. After experiencing the elation of helping Nyguen walk again and the anger of watching so many needlessly suffer in Vietnam, I decided that I wanted to help poor people with fractures in developing countries.

This book describes the journey of SIGN Fracture Care International. SIGN, for short, has evolved into an orthopaedic humanitarian aid organization that assists local surgeons in treating impoverished people in developing countries. SIGN supplies surgical

---

[1]   Gosselin, Richard A.; Spiegel, David A.; Coughlin, Richard Coughlin; and Zirkle, Lewis G. "Injuries: the neglected burden in developing countries." WHO. April 04, 2009. Accessed April 13, 2017. http://www.who.int/bulletin/volumes/87/4/08-052290/en/.

implants and training to orthopaedic surgeons at no cost, provided that the patient is not charged for the implants. SIGN has started programs in more than 300 hospitals throughout 50 developing countries as of 2017. The patient is the focus of everything we do. The majority of the SIGN Surgery is done by local surgeons.

More than 5,000 SIGN Surgeons now use the SIGN System to treat fractures largely caused by road traffic accidents. Since 1999, more than 200,000 patients have been treated with the SIGN System. SIGN helps surgeons in developing countries establish programs where the need for fracture care is most severe. We all share a vision of creating equality of fracture care for all patients.

In this book, I describe the beginnings of SIGN and its culture. I explain how we evolved from a few surgeons trying to develop an implant to a global organization devoted to improving fracture care. We are not a hierarchy and we all share ideas about treatment, education, and implants. I discuss the agony and the ecstasy of providing care to severely injured patients. I discuss the mistakes I made and knowledge gained. Finally, I share my hopes and dreams for the future of SIGN Fracture Care International.

Chapter 2

Equality

The vision of SIGN Fracture Care International is "creating equality of fracture care throughout the world." I first learned the value and impact of creating equality from my father. Dad was a big man in many ways. He stood 6 foot 5 inches tall. He played football at Ohio State University. Football taught my father the importance of fairness and treating people equally regardless of their background.

It was in North Carolina, however, where my father demonstrated how important equality was to him. He was employed by General Electric, and they assigned him to supervise the building and administration of a new factory. The 1956 building codes required the construction of four bathrooms on each floor, so people of different sexes and colors could do their business in separate spaces. At that time, North Carolina was segregated. Blacks and whites were divided by Jim Crow laws mandating that public facilities be "separate but equal." The reality of these laws usually meant that facilities for blacks were inferior and unequal to those built for whites. My father authorized construction of four bathrooms, but he only opened two of them, designated Men and Women. One day, Luther Hodges, governor of North Carolina, came to visit the newly constructed factory. He noted with satisfaction that the building complied with the manufacturing codes. He appeared not to pay attention to the signs on the bathrooms, although Dad noticed he scrutinized them.

When he left, Gov. Hodges told my father, "Lew, you're doing a good job."

I credit my dad with giving me another opportunity to learn about equality. He found me a summer job stacking lumber at Yount Lumber Company when I was still a teenager. I was the only white laborer assigned to stacking green lumber, and I quickly made friends with the African-American laborers. Nothing brings people closer together than working toward a common goal. We had to work together because freshly cut lumber is very heavy and the boards were often perilously stacked as high as 20 feet. Together, we would ride through town laughing and joking in the back of the lumber truck. On Saturday night, my new friends placed their stereos beside the road and turned up the volume to play loud music. We danced in the street and had a fine time. Our friendship overrode segregation.

Each summer I was assigned to a different job at Yount Lumber and soon became a carpenter. I continued to spend my lunch hours eating with my African-American friends. I seemed to have more in common with them than I had with the other workers. Perhaps this commonality was simply that we had all worked hard as a team stacking green lumber. I appreciated that these men treated me as an equal, just as I treated them.

I enjoyed working with wood and building things and wanted a career as a carpenter, but my mother stated firmly I should go to college. I applied and was accepted at Davidson College, 29 miles away from home. I discovered a vast difference between what I had learned in high school and what the other students who attended private high schools and better public high schools had learned. My preparation for college was inferior to many of my college peers. My grades were below average at Davidson, and I was in constant fear of failing. I gained an appreciation of how stressful it can be when you did not have the opportunities afforded others.

Physical activity had always provided relief from stress, so I went out for football, even though I had played only two years in high school. I tried hard, learned the rules, and made the varsity team my junior year. This success on the gridiron relieved my sense of inferiority that I felt from my poor scholastic preparation for college.

I became good friends with my roommate and the two boys across the hall at Davidson. They were all determined to go to medical school after college, so I took the same classes they did. After completing college, I applied to enter medical school. I interviewed at Duke University Medical Center in Durham, North Carolina, and was accepted.

I will always be grateful to Duke for admitting me, as I felt very inadequate academically. I am also grateful to Duke for emphasizing a culture of equality to their medical students. Our professors demanded that physicians treat all patients with dignity and be their advocate. Patients being addressed as "Mr." or "Mrs." followed by their last name, for example, showed respect. The professors also demanded that we students learn about what the conditions were like in the hometowns of our patients, no matter where they lived. They stressed that knowing about the patients' environment helped to facilitate diagnosing and treating their problems. The demands of my mentors at Duke further ingrained my belief in equality for all people. We may not be born with the same mental and physical abilities, the same opportunities, or we may not live in the same conditions, but we all have the same spark of humanity.

My grades at Duke during the first two years (which were spent learning biology and biochemistry) were average, but they improved substantially during my third year when we began to see patients. I now appreciated that learning these facts and formulas about chemistry and physiology, which seemed irrelevant in my first years of medical school, formed the basis for helping my patients. I decided that even though it might take me six years to learn what my class-mates learned in four years, I must learn and develop the skills to provide the best medical care possible for all patients.

Dr. Lenox Baker was chief of orthopaedic surgery at Duke and known for being frank and demanding, and was prone to tirades when residents displeased him. One day during my first year of medical school, I was walking down the hall when I heard someone behind me yell, "Hey, boy!" I looked around and realized that Dr. Baker, whom I only knew by reputation, was yelling at me. He told me that the next day he would operate on my brother, Fred, who played football at Duke, and he asked if I would like to scrub with him. I told him I had never been in surgery. He said he would teach me and told me to meet him at seven o'clock the next morning.

When I arrived, Dr. Baker took me into the faculty room and told me to put my clothes in the locker of the medical school dean, a neurosurgeon. I was apprehensive about this as I imagined the dean might want to use his locker. Besides, my clothes were not fashionable. My mother bought all my clothes and had purchased orange shoes that were a little long and curled up in front. I assume their biggest asset to my mother was their sale price. When she handed them over to me, she had assured me that someday they would be the fashion. Fortunately, the dean never found my funny shoes or my clothes in his locker that day.

Dr. Baker and I proceeded to the operating room where an ortho-paedic resident was washing and placing drapes around my brother's leg. Dr. Baker corrected him so loudly and with such vigor that the resident's knees began to shake. We turned to scrubbing our hands and arms, and Dr. Baker helped me into a surgical gown and sent the orthopaedic resident to the other side of the table so he could show me how to remove my brother's knee cartilage. Watching Dr. Baker in surgery was very exciting for me. The case lasted 60 minutes, but I felt that it lasted only five minutes. I admired the combination of Dr. Baker's intellectual and physical skill.

After the surgery, Dr. Baker became my mentor. During my third year in medical school, I spent my surgical rotation taking the place of an orthopaedic resident—seeing patients on the ward, in the clinic, and assisting in surgery. After my third year, Dr. Baker asked me what residency I would like to pursue, and I told him I wanted to be an orthopaedic surgeon. "Fine, boy," he said. "I'll make you a resident after your internship." I was surprised. The standard progression of surgical training was to take a year of general surgery after internship, to prepare for surgical specialization, such as orthopaedic surgery. The fact that he accepted me into the program after only one year of internship, allowing me to skip an extra year of general surgery training, had far-reaching consequences for me when I was drafted into the Army in 1968. The Army designated me as an orthopaedic surgeon rather than general medical officer since I had one year of orthopaedic training.

As I got to know Dr. Baker, I realized that while he was gruff to orthopaedic residents, he was very courteous and compassionate to his patients, especially disabled children. He started the Crippled Children's Hospital of North Carolina, a pioneer hospital for treating children with cerebral palsy. Dr. Baker became their advocate. He taught me by example that equality means not just treating all patients with respect, but also providing special care to those patients who did not consider themselves equal to others. He took residents to outlying communities to treat the disabled children of parents who could not afford to travel to the hospital. He taught me that sometimes we have to spend more time and resources to help patients with disabilities. A good doctor has to make up for the inequality that some patients suffer.

I have learned so much about equality and empathy and compassion from my father and Dr. Baker. They championed the weak and the underserved. These mentors were not guided by conventional wisdom; they made decisions based on what they believed was right, and they were both tough, but tender to the disadvantaged. They always "provided a hand down," an expression I learned much later in Haiti from Dr. George Dyer, chief of Harvard's orthopaedic training program. Dr. Dyer used the metaphor to explain that all of us, somewhere in our careers, are recipients of an extended arm from others.

I met my wife Sara in medical school. She was a year ahead of me at Duke. Her grades were at the top of her class. She was interested in pediatrics and admired those that champion the weak and underserved. She subspecialized in developmental behavior, which was a new specialty at the time. Her patients all needed a "hand down" because many were developmentally delayed or had other emotional problems.

The Army drafted me in 1968 and gave me the option of going to Vietnam my first or second year of service. I chose my first year because Sara and I had two young daughters. Sara was in her final year of pediatric residency. My brother, Fred, lived with us and could assist Sara in caring for our daughters. I knew they would all be in good hands, especially when Dr. Baker also said he'd look after them. Sara is quiet and unassuming; she is pint-sized but mighty and conquers adversity with aplomb. During my absence, she exhibited great resilience, juggling her pediatric residency duties and caring for our two daughters.

Chapter 3

The Army

I arrived in Bien Hoa, Vietnam, on a transport plane carrying fresh US troops just as the Viet Cong blew up the ammo dump near the landing field there. We had disembarked the plane and were being taken to temporary quarters. When a mushroom-shaped cloud arose, an orthopaedic surgeon who'd been on the flight yelled, "It's a nuke!" and dove under a bed. As he dove for cover, he become entangled with a large anesthetist who also sought protection under the same bed. As the rest of us extracted these two from their embarrassing position, I learned that the orthopaedic surgeon would be my chief at the 93rd Evacuation Hospital (93rd Evac).

A month later, we staged a ceremony where we celebrated his nuke exclamation and bed dive. We painted a flak jacket yellow and labeled it "Chicken of the Month." That was my first experience with laughter mixed with war. I have to say that war is no comedy. It is devastating for everyone on all sides of the fighting. However, the Army taught me that a little bit of humor could go a long way toward coping with the stress and horror of combat. My comrades and I played our share of pranks on each other and our officers. Laughter has healing properties, but we never forgot we were there to heal others. Both the orthopaedic surgeon and the anesthetist later earned our respect as excellent physicians. One of my assignments in Vietnam was to be the commanding officer of a K team. It was a nebulous assignment and I still do not know what a K team is. I was to serve as liaison with the helicopter crews called to pick up the wounded and fly them to the 93rd Evac.

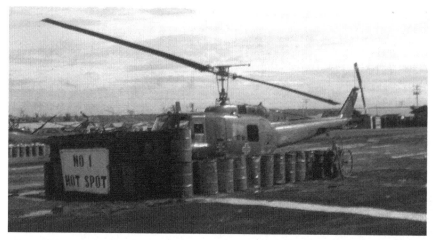

US military helicopter pilots and crews risked their lives to evacuate all wounded people—soldiers and civilians.

While serving as their liaison, I developed the highest respect for the pilots and crew who risked their lives to evacuate all the wounded from the battlefield—US military, Vietnamese military, and Vietnamese civilians. When the wounded arrived at the 93rd Evac, we were to treat US military and send wounded Vietnamese civilians to another hospital. I visited the other hospital and felt that the facility and personnel were not equipped to care for severely wounded patients. I believed that these injured Vietnamese civilians, who had no stake in the conflict but suffered from the fighting, were victims. They deserved optimal care. They deserved care equal to what we were giving to the wounded US military.

One of the wounded US fighters was Col. Joe Fix, a well-known soldier and commander of US forces during the battle of Dak To. Generals Westmoreland and Abrams, the commanders of all US forces in Vietnam, visited Col. Fix almost daily. During their visits, Col. Fix praised my care of his fractured leg, even though I didn't think my treatment was anything spectacular. Nevertheless, I took advantage of his accolades to ask Col. Joseph Kovaric, commanding officer of the 93rd Evac, if I could treat the wounded Vietnamese civilians in our hospital. My request prompted several discussions between Col. Kovaric and the generals.

Permission was granted to treat Vietnamese civilians at our hospital. One entire Quonset hut was assigned as a ward for injured Vietnamese civilians. Our hospital was a collection of Quonset huts because the Viet Cong could disable an entire inflatable MASH Hospital by simply shooting the generator that kept the tents inflated.

Despite getting my commanders to approve our efforts to take care of both US military and Vietnamese civilian casualties, we had to treat each group differently. It was against Army regulations to use metal implants to fix fractures in wounded US soldiers. The medical leaders of our armed forces were concerned about the potential for infection when broken bones were treated in facilities that were close to the battleground. The military patients were evacuated to Japan or the United States for more definitive care. We provided definitive fracture care to Vietnamese civilians, however, because they had nowhere else to go. We used metal implants to stabilize their fractures, and they healed without infection. Surgeons along the evacuation chain and friends in the US sent me a variety of rods, plates, and screws to treat the civilians. Nurses and anesthesiologists worked overtime so we could operate on them after we had finished treating the injured soldiers. I learned that people could be very kind when they are given a chance. The patients were treated long enough for the fracture to heal so they could walk on crutches. After we had begun treating Vietnamese patients, we noted that the rocket attacks directed at our hospital stopped. We found out later that the 93rd Evac was near the end of the Ho Chi Minh Trail, an important supply route for the Viet Cong fighters who were battling the US and their South Vietnamese allies. I like to think that the Viet Cong suspended their attacks on our hospital because they knew we were doing a good job treating Vietnamese civilians.

In order to understand more about war from the viewpoint of the soldier, I asked my commanding officer if I could take off my rank, go through jungle training with the 101st Airborne Division, and then participate in missions. After I received permission to join the fighters of the 101st Airborne, I discovered that I was a very poor shot with an M-16 rifle, and I was not especially good at marching in unison with the other soldiers. The sergeants tolerated my ineptitude.

One night we were ordered to walk night patrol through the jungle. We came to a halt when one of the soldiers told the sergeant that he had lost his pack. The sergeant berated him very loudly. I was concerned about the noise because I was sure every tree around us was hiding an enemy sniper. The soldier, probably no more than 16 years old, began to cry. His immature brain couldn't handle the trauma of war combined with the sergeant's berating. I knew the human brain does not mature until age 26, and a thought occurred to me: This is a war fought by immature adolescents! I did not participate in more missions with the 101st Airborne. My epiphany about how this war was really fought transformed into a growing rage.

Fortunately, a little humor helped reduce my anger. One night each week, we watched the weekly comedy and variety show *Laugh-In* on a 12-inch television set. We tried to turn the recreational evening into a vacation, and several surgeons set up beach chairs. It was our night to forget the war.

Humor was an antidote. I have read that it is also a form of rebellion. Sometimes we relieved the stress of war by playing pranks. We were told not to use a flashlight at night when we used the latrine. One of the administrative officers, coincidentally a urologist, insisted on using a flashlight whenever he visited the facilities. Every night as he sat there, his light projected from the latrine. One night we surrounded the latrine and threw rocks on its tin roof. Just before the rocks landed, we yelled "Incoming!" which meant there was an incoming rocket attack. We could see his flashlight beam bouncing erratically in the dark as he ran out of the latrine. After that, we didn't see any more lights in the latrine.

The targets of our pranks were not random. Most of the regular Army surgeons were excellent doctors whom we respected because they garnered our admiration with their actions. We believed that authority was earned rather than bestowed by insignia on a uniform. Those who attempted to gain respect simply because of their rank were the subjects of our pranks. My experiences in Vietnam taught me the importance of judging people based on ability rather than title. I have tried to incorporate this lesson into the SIGN Philosophy. SIGN is not a hierarchical organization.

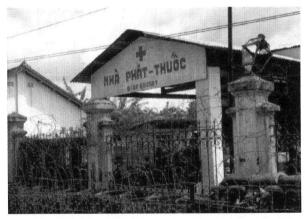

The war disrupted medical care for Vietnamese civilians.

I continued to spend long hours operating on US Army troops and Vietnamese civilians, but I wanted to do more. I asked Col. Kovaric if I could be the Civil Actions Officer for the hospital and was granted permission. The traditional Army outreach activity was called

MEDCAP, which included traveling by convoy to countryside clinics to treat civilians. The civilian medical establishment in Vietnam had collapsed during the war, and barbed wire surrounded most of the clinics. On my travels, I observed that many patients simply wanted cough drops and dental care. Our most important contribution was pulling rotten teeth. Despite the successes, none of our treatments were easy as most of the patients were suspicious of any American in a uniform.

After one of our jeeps was booby-trapped with a hidden bomb during a MEDCAP operation, I decided there must be a better way to help the Vietnamese civilians. I found an orphanage staffed by North Vietnamese nuns. Most of the work I did in the orphanage included general health, wellness, and treatment of infections. My wife Sara advised me about the pediatric and public health treatment of both individual patients and the orphanage. The nuns worked under difficult conditions and were very caring.

One day the nuns told me that the Viet Cong had entered the back of the orphanage and were looking for me. I left immediately through the front door. When I came back a few days later to thank the nuns for the warning, they were gone. I was despondent. Their disappearance was another inequity, and I had caused it. I carried the burden of the nuns' disappearance for many years. Twenty-five years later, I was sitting in a church in Vietnam when I saw a picture of Jesus and his sheep. Under the painting were the words: "Feed my sheep." I remembered that the Bible teaches that Jesus looks after his sheep, and I finally felt relief. The nuns were in His hands.

Memories of war never disappear. These memories are a combination of nostalgia for the friendships forged under pressure, the adrenaline rush of fearing for your life, and the dread and terror of seeing people needlessly suffer and die. These memories can cause veterans of war to crave stimulation that fills a void left by battle or they can make other veterans struggle to function in the mundane life of the civilian world. Just when you think these memories are buried, something pulls them back.

The movie *Whiskey Tango Foxtrot* accurately depicts people bound together in times of conflict who develop feelings of brotherhood. After their tours ended, some of the movie's characters remained in Afghanistan because of those tribal bonds. Some people miss the adrenaline of conflict and look for other ways to satisfy the craving. Some people have trouble reintegrating into civilian life. Memories of wartime experience are never far from the surface. I visited Afghanistan for the third time in November 2015 and stayed in a military hospital. Helicopters began arriving at five o'clock in the morning, carrying the wounded. I tossed and turned as memories of Vietnam resurfaced.

In the end, it is good to retain access to our memories. The National Archives Building in Washington, D.C., bears the inscription: "What is past is prologue." I think that means we need to reflect on our past, so we can learn from it. *Stripping Bare the Body: Politics, Violence, War*, a book by Mark Danner, chronicles the history of politics in Haiti, the Balkans, Iraq, and the United States. Danner notes that "stripping bare the body" means we must look at the heart and reason for our actions. We must evaluate our role as a country and as individuals in conflicts around the world. We need to learn from our mistakes. There were many outcries about the United States and early opposition to the successful slave rebellion in Haiti that led to its independence in 1804. The criticism came because, instead of supporting the liberated slaves who founded the new nation, the United States failed to formally recognize the country and actively tried to destroy it. Danner's retrospective study emphasizes that we must evaluate our past, and outcries alone do not stop injustice. Real change demands something more than words.

Words are the shadows of actions. If we want to change things, we must act.

We seem fascinated by conflict from a distance, but we often fail to show empathy for the victims of the conflict. When we ignore the victims, we are moral idiots. Vietnam taught me the importance of empathy. It made me realize the power of humor and the significance of basing respect on the merit of one's actions rather than the rank on their uniform. It made me have faith in those who sacrifice to ease the burden of those who suffer. My recollections of the war are bittersweet, but these memories have forged a determination to do more than criticize an injustice. I now know I need to act in order to change something for the better.

Chapter 4

The Indonesian Man in the Bed

In 1969, I left Vietnam and returned to the United States. I was assigned to Fitzsimmons Army Hospital in Aurora, CO. My chief at Fitzsimmons Army Hospital, Col. Bill Burkhalter, was an original thinker not bound by conventional wisdom. He sought unique solutions for problems. You could almost see a light bulb turn on over his head as an idea was emerging. When the insight struck, his face would become red, his blue eyes would bulge, and he would pace around the room as he explained his idea.

I saw this happen when we were treating a patient that had a very severe leg injury. Swelling of the tissues in the damaged extremity had caused enough pressure in the patient's leg muscles to compromise their blood supply. If this condition, known as compartment syndrome, had been diagnosed earlier, we would have reduced the pressure by cutting open the fascia around the leg muscles and restoring the blood flow. It was, unfortunately, too late for our patient. By the time we made the diagnosis, his muscles were dead from lack of adequate perfusion. The standard treatment for patients who have necrotic leg muscles is amputation. The dead tissue must be removed before it becomes infected and threatens the life of the patient. Our patient, however, still had sensation at the bottom of his foot. Dr. Burkhalter's light bulb turned on. He reasoned that this patient would have better function using a leg with withered muscles and a foot with feeling than trying to live with a prosthesis devoid of feeling. Dr. Burkhalter was right, and our patient was eventually able to walk again on his atrophied but sensate leg. I was fortunate to be exposed to mentors like Dr. Burkhalter, Dr. Baker, and my other teachers at Duke. They showed respect for all people. They sought the optimum care for all. They were problem solvers. They weren't afraid to act on the inspiration of an idea in order to improve a bad situation.

While I was in Vietnam, Dr. Baker retired. Dr. J. Leonard Goldner was appointed as the chief of the orthopaedic surgery program at Duke University School of Medicine. I wrote Dr. Goldner, telling him that I was ready to return to Duke after discharge from the Army. He said I could come back, but Duke did not give credit for service in the Army toward completion of its orthopaedic program. This was disappointing, as I had learned a great deal of orthopaedic surgery during my service in Vietnam. I was also learning a great deal of orthopaedics from Dr. Burkhalter and the Army consultants. Fortune smiled on me when Dr. Burkhalter said he would recommend me for an orthopaedic resident opening at Letterman Army Hospital in San Francisco, CA. This residency included spending a year at the Los Angeles Shriners Hospital for Children. I accepted.

My rotation at Los Angeles Shriners Hospital for Children was one of the highlights of my training in the Army. Many of the patients at Shriners were from Mexico and presented with deformities caused by childhood polio. Dr. Will Weston worked at the Shriners Hospital and he was another original thinker. Together we treated many patients with dwarfism and polio. We surgically corrected a number of unusual deformities. We spent every third night in the hospital. During night rounds, the patients at Shriners taught me Spanish. At the time, I thought they laughed at my pronunciation. I learned later that the words they taught me were off-color. I realized these patients were using humor the way I had during my days in Vietnam. It was a way for them to cope and to rebel against injustice.

Once again I was able to apply lessons I learned at Duke about the value of understanding the patient's point of view. I knew their laughter wasn't mockery; it was a form of therapy. While in Los Angeles in 1970, I visited Dr. Charles Bechtel, another innovative surgeon. Bechtel was a pioneer of hip replacement surgery, which was a relatively new operation that had started in England. He modified the English technique, designed implants to fit his modification, and held frequent teaching courses dedicated to total hip arthroplasty. He invited me to join him for three months.

Dr. Bechtel devised his own original way to look at hip radiographs. He would take x-rays of the patients' hips from different angles and put them side by side on the view box. He would then cross his eyes and see a 3-D image of the hip. I was never able to do this despite staring cross-eyed at a large number of x-rays. Dr. Bechtel and I ate breakfast together every morning in the hospital and discussed new ideas. We scrubbed together on total hip surgery procedures. Many orthopaedic surgeons traveled to Los Angeles in order to watch him perform hip replacement. I couldn't believe these visitors, who often were noted surgeons and authored articles I had read, were now asking me questions about hip surgery!

My next assignment was Fort Ord, on Monterey Bay in California. One of our consultants was Dr. L.D. Howard, a pioneer of hand surgery. He was retired, lived in a nearby town, and drove to Fort Ord Hospital one day every week. We always met him at the entrance and escorted him to the operating room. He was a very good surgeon and could repair hand tendons skillfully and rapidly. There are many vital structures in the hand. I watched Dr. Howard very carefully move them to the side to expose the damaged tendon. He never wasted motion when he was operating.

I learned a great deal from Dr. Howard. His skill in the operating room demonstrated that procedural memory may fade, but it returns rapidly when it is needed. Procedural memory, or unconscious motor memory, is like riding a bicycle. Once you learn, the process stays with you. If, after many years of not riding, you are given the opportunity to ride again, the skill quickly returns.

Psychologist K. Anders Ericsson asserts that this type of memory must be renewed by deliberate practice. In his recent book, *Peak*, Ericsson maintains that after six months, procedural memory skills wane and practice is necessary to bring them up to speed. This is especially true when it comes to surgery. I travel to SIGN Programs at least every four months to keep my surgical skills sharp. SIGN now incorporates this principle of procedural memory in our educational materials. We provide a written manual so doctors can read and learn about the implant. But we also have designed simulators so surgeons can practice the more difficult parts of SIGN Surgery. Some surgeons develop the procedural or motor memory faster than others do. Ericsson notes that knowledge does not equate to surgical skill. Surgeons must practice with their hands as well as their minds in order to improve surgical skills.

Fort Ord was an infantry training facility and, therefore, strict Army regulations governed our conduct. My wife Sara never liked Army life. Her father had spent five years stationed in the Aleutian Islands during World War II. He never talked about his time there, but his absence had a big influence on his children. Sara grew up missing her dad and resenting military protocol. She took the combat patch off my Army uniform and sewed a Snoopy patch in its place. The canine patch made quite a hit with the enlisted men, and they soon began to sew funny patches on their uniforms. No one complained!

I remained at Fort Ord for one year to complete my Army obligation. I am indebted to the Army for giving me an opportunity to learn surgery from many mentors. During my annual leave at Fort Ord, Sara and I went to Indonesia with CARE MEDICO. Dr. Tom Dooley, a surgeon who worked in Southeast Asia treating the poor, established CARE MEDICO. It was a model of an effective volunteer effort that served the developing world.

In 1970, I helped Dr. Soelarto, the sole Indonesian orthopaedic surgeon, during my leave of duty from the Army. Together we started four training programs in different parts of Indonesia. Our plan included delivering didactic lectures about orthopaedic surgery and distributing donated implants and orthopaedic equipment. Over the years, I was able to return annually to Indonesia for several weeks each year. More than 25 years later, in 1996, while visiting one of the Indonesian surgeons who was my student during my days with CARE MEDICO, I realized that the concept of lectures plus donation of random equipment was not effective. Much of the donated equipment never arrived where it was supposed to go, and when it did reach the correct destination, it was often unusable or obsolete. I was beginning to realize that my efforts had been inadequate.

The light bulb came on over my head when I saw a man lying in bed and heard his story. He had pins in his bones attached to weights pulling on the pins. He was in traction, a common way to treat fractures of the femur. Most of the patients on the ward had traction weights extending from pins in their legs. Unfortunately, many of these fractures healed poorly or didn't heal at all. That's what happened to the man in the bed.

The patient was very depressed because he had been in bed for three years waiting for his fracture to heal. His family had stopped coming to visit because they could not afford the daily hospital charges. An x-ray, taken many months before, showed that the ends of his fractured bones were far apart. The surgeon and I knew the man's fracture would never heal. Both ends of a fracture like his must be brought together and held securely with a metal implant in order to heal. I asked the surgeon why he hadn't done surgery to treat the man's fracture. I reminded him that I had lectured to him about this type of surgery years ago when he was my student.

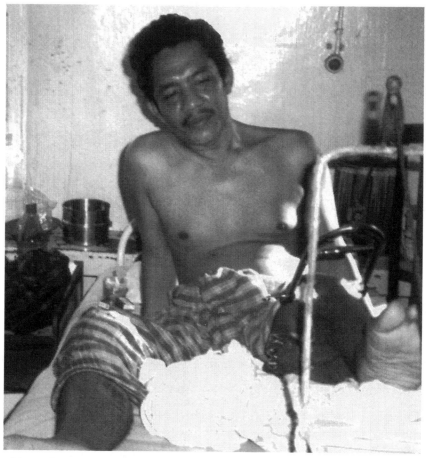

This Indonesian man in the bed inspired the SIGN Model—educating doctors and providing appropriate implants.

He said that he had remembered my lectures, but his patient could not afford the implants to treat his fracture. He explained that, in addition, the implants we sent to Indonesia could not be used because they were designed to be inserted with power tools and instant x-rays in the operating room. His hospital had power surges and the surgeons could not use equipment that required electricity. He also stated that the implants we sent were not practical because they did not contain a full set of sizes that fit his patients' bones. I realized with a sinking heart that I had wasted years of effort in Indonesia because I had not validated my regimen of lectures, surgery, and providing donated implants. I never confirmed whether we actually supplied implants that allowed surgeons to perform the procedures we were trying to teach them. The treatment concepts I had taught were useful but the equipment was designed for conditions in the developed world, not the operating rooms of Indonesia.

The lesson I learned was that implants and instruments must be donated to treat the poor who cannot pay for the implants. The implants, in addition, must be suitable for the conditions in their operating rooms. The implants should not require the use of power tools when there is no reliable electricity. They cannot depend on a sophisticated x-ray machine to guide their insertion during surgery when the hospital can't afford to buy or maintain such equipment. The implants, furthermore, must be provided in different sizes that fit the bones of the patients in that part of the world.

I also learned the value of validation of our efforts. If we are going to take the trouble to organize teaching sessions, solicit donations, design implants, and ship them overseas, we have to make sure that those sessions, that money, and the implants reach the people who can use them the most. As SIGN grew, I made it a point to remember that poor Indonesian man who languished in a bed for three years waiting for his broken leg to heal. Today his photograph hangs on the walls of SIGN Headquarters as a reminder and an incentive for the SIGN Staff. I hope this picture makes SIGN Surgeons ask: "Will my treatment decision get the patient out of bed?" I also hope that the photo of the Indonesian man in bed motivates our surgeons to ask themselves: "How many more patients will my decisions help get out of bed?"

I changed my focus from Indonesia to Vietnam in 1985 when I received three calls in one day. Each caller had a reason for asking me to return to Vietnam. One was a man who told me that he had been a scout with the US Special Forces when his helicopter was shot down. He sustained severe wounds to his leg and arm and lay in the jungle for three weeks before he was rescued and taken to the 93rd Evacuation Hospital. His wounds had become infected and his arm and leg were amputated to save his life. Somehow, he knew I was the surgeon who had cared for him and performed his life-saving surgery. He asked me to return to Vietnam to help his people, who were now suffering injuries like he had experienced. How could I refuse?

The second caller hailed from Houston, TX. He had immigrated to the US after the American forces withdrew from South Vietnam. He knew how I had helped local casualties and was aware how the Vietnamese continued to need help treating fractures.

The third caller was a Vietnamese woman named Tammy Crisp who settled in my hometown, Richland, WA. Her nephew was still in Vietnam. He had his severely fractured leg treated in traction there. He was unable to walk because his leg had healed in a poor position. She asked if there was any way I could help him walk again.

All of these callers were very insistent and convincing.

In order to get permission to enter Vietnam in 1985, I traveled to Bangkok, Thailand, and went to the Vietnamese embassy there to get a visa. Day after day, they kept telling me to come back. Then I heard I could get a visa on the black market. I managed to find someone who would sell me the visa I needed. I can still smell the garlic on the breath of the person waiting in line behind me when he yelled at my visa salesman: "Hey, my friend bought a visa from you three months ago and was supposed to have been home six weeks ago, but he has not returned. What happened?"

When I arrived in Vietnam on the plane there was a great deal of emotion and crying at the airport. The majority of passengers were Vietnamese who had escaped the war and were now returning to see their families. Upon arrival, I could not find my bags, which contained orthopaedic implants. I looked behind the airport and found my duffel bags leaning against the wall. I was no longer in the Army, but I used my US Army duffel bags labeled "Cpt. L. Zirkle." I realized then that traveling with my old military duffel bags was a mistake. The Vietnamese officials at the airport thought I was a CIA agent. After I found my bags, a woman called me by name and told me she would take me to a hospital. I found out later she was a friend of Tammy Crisp, the woman who had summoned me from my hometown. The customs officers were not only suspicious of the appearance of my bags, they were also skeptical about the implants I transported inside them. This woman fluently lobbied on my behalf, convincing the officials to let me in the country.

She took me to a hospital in Song Be province, where more puzzled officials directed me to rest from my journey in a hospital room. The beginning of this trip was far from a vacation. I couldn't sleep because people visited my room at all hours of the day and night for three days. The clanging of metal next door was extremely loud. To top it off, the room was filled with buzzing mosquitoes. I tried to spray the insects, but when I pushed the button, the can exploded with a boom, leaving my room filled with a fog of repellent and many people who had rushed in.

After three days of fighting mosquitoes in my room, the hospital officials took me to another space with approximately 50 patients dressed in white gowns. The patients had assorted orthopaedic injuries and limb deformities from polio. It took me several days to examine them all and provide treatment suggestions. Soon after this, I was led to another building in very poor repair. I realized that this was their surgery facility when I saw an oxygen tank with hoses going into two rooms. Inside one of the rooms was a patient I had seen during my previous consultations. He was now asleep on the operating table, unconscious from breathing the fumes of ether dropped on a mask held under his face. The fumes from ether anesthesia can be very dangerous because they are flammable. The surgeon, therefore, cannot use an electrocautery, an important tool to ligate bleeding vessels during the operation. The spark from the instrument can ignite the ether fumes and blow up the operating room and everyone inside it. The patient had sustained a femur fracture in the war that Vietnam was fighting with neighboring Cambodia. The hospital director ordered the chief of orthopaedic surgery to operate on the patient's femur.

As soon as he made the incision, I realized that this chief of orthopaedic surgery had no clue how to do the operation. Nor did he understand English. He had learned surgery in the Cu Chi tunnels, a network of clandestine passageways connecting North and South Vietnam. The North Vietnamese used caverns within the tunnels as hospitals to treat their wounded soldiers. The operation was awkward, but we proceeded by communicating with grunts and hand gestures. I tried to be as tactful as possible as we placed the bone fragments back together and stabilized them with orthopaedic plates from my duffel bag. This surgery was the first of a steady stream of operations that followed my initial consultations.

Tammy Crisp's nephew was one of those many patients. As I mentioned, many of the patients suffered from polio deformities, and I corrected them using the principles I had learned at Los Angeles Shriners Hospital. One patient was a girl with contracted neck muscles that deformed her face. Her operation required lengthening the muscles while moving vital neck vessels out of my way. The ether anesthesia prevented me from using a cautery to control bleeding that occurs from mobilizing these vessels. The surgery, therefore, was more challenging and difficult than usual. Fortunately, the operation went well. Much later when I was back home doing difficult surgeries in Richland, I would recall this Vietnamese girl's neck surgery and I would, simultaneously, hear the words of my partner of many years, Dr. Ted Samsell: "We don't ask that this operation be easy, just possible."

While in Vietnam I kept my precious airline tickets safely stored in a pouch around my waist. After three weeks of sweating in the operating room, they were saturated and faded. I was able to decipher that it was time to go home. I told the hospital director that I had to go. He told me that I could not go because there were more patients who needed surgery. I explained that if I missed my flight I would never return to Vietnam. When he realized that I made a pledge to come back, he found the only car in the province—a Yugo—and we started for the airport. None of us was sure how to drive this car. As we accelerated to go up a steep rise over a bridge, the Yugo hit a bump, and the engine stopped. A local man who knew how to fix the Yugo appeared, fixed the car, and we proceeded to the airport just in time for my flight back to Bangkok.

I returned to Vietnam nearly every year for the next 20 years. During this time, I gained respect for how the Vietnamese surgeons were innovative and eager to learn. In 1990, I sent a container of books to a hospital in Ho Chi Minh City. The administrators responded by building a library on top of the hospital. We bonded with a shared interest in using orthopaedic surgery to alleviate suffering.

In 1991, I helped organized a conference for surgeons from both North and South Vietnam. Many of these surgeons had never met. They had been enemies during the war. The younger surgeons from

North Vietnam had trained in hospitals in the Cu Chi tunnels. The older surgeons from North Vietnam had trained in medical schools that were destroyed by bombing. Most of the surgeons from the South had been to medical school, but they had been forced by their North Vietnamese vanquishers to spend years in reeducation camps after the war. The conference was successful despite these differences and some dogmatic statements about patient care asserted by both sides. When the conference concluded, all of us rode motorcycles to a boat that had been converted to a restaurant. We drank a lot of beer and someone started singing. Others joined in. The chief of orthopaedic surgery at Stanford Medical Center in California, Dr. Don Nagel, contributed an old sailor's ditty. Soon the boatload of surgeons were singing. We all were united by beer and interest in orthopaedic surgery.

Over the years, the Vietnamese surgeons learned to speak English and we became good friends. Dr. Han Khoi Quang, a surgeon trained in the Cu Chi tunnel hospitals, and I became especially close. I think we admired each other's confidence and knowledge of fracture care but frequently we disagreed about orthopaedic surgery. Sometimes these disagreements became loud. Looking back, he was right more times than I was, and Dr. Quang made many pioneering observations about SIGN Techniques and Indications. He demonstrated and explained how we could use the SIGN Nail without modification by placing it through the upper end of the femur. My trips to Vietnam and vigorous discussions with Dr. Quang showed me that diversity of opinion coupled with friendship is important for innovation.

On one trip, I was invited to a meeting at the home of a surgeon in Ho Chi Minh City. He took a risk by inviting me because the government forbade associating with Americans. I was invited to look in his upstairs closet. Inside, I saw a screw machine he used to put threads on pins for treating hip fractures. Ingenuity and persistence are characteristic of the Vietnamese people.

On another visit to Ho Chi Minh City in 2002, an ambulance driver met me at the airport and drove me to Song Be Hospital. Sirens wailed and lights flashed all the way, and my ears were ringing. When we arrived, I was taken to see a 15-year-old girl who had been hit by a motorcycle. She had fractures of her femur and tibia, with a big defect in her muscles and skin that exposed the tibia. She also had torn a major artery in her leg. We put SIGN Nails into her femur and tibia and repaired the artery. We then transferred her to Dr. Tuan in Ho Chi Minh City, who covered the bone with soft tissues. She healed from her wound and fractures. Her results could not have been better if treated anywhere else in the world at that time.

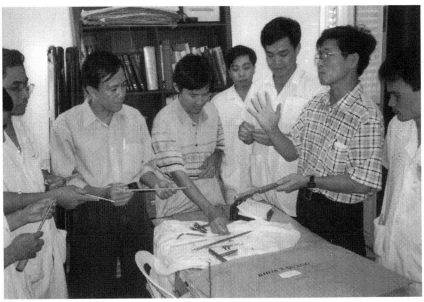

Vietnamese surgeons provided invaluable feedback to our early designs of SIGN Equipment.

Dr. Tuan now teaches soft tissue surgery and does research in Ho Chi Minh City. He also was an early pioneer of SIGN Surgery.

We had many good times together doing SIGN Surgery as we developed new ideas and implants. When he visited SIGN in May 2016, we fell back into our former routine of animated discussions.

Road traffic accidents in Vietnam continued to increase, not only the number of fractures but also head injuries. Bicycles and vehicles in Vietnam swirled on the streets like schools of fish. One day I stood on the corner of a busy street in Hanoi wondering how to get across the road through these motorcycles. My ego was punctured when I saw a woman slowly moving across the street. She was blind.

To make matters worse, no one wore helmets. When a motorcycle driver or rider suffered a blow to the unprotected head, orthopaedic surgeons drilled holes in the skull in order to release the blood that was pushing on the victim's brain. I shipped a container full of bicycle helmets to Vietnam. Dr. Long, the chief of orthopaedics at Cho Ray Hospital, took charge of these helmets and made a rule that no hospital employee could enter the hospital parking lot without wearing one. I remember one day that we were sitting on his motorcycle discussing this rule when I noticed that his helmet was on backward. He wasn't happy to be corrected. His example, however, had a positive effect. Eventually, the Vietnamese government required all motorcyclists to wear a helmet while riding on a highway.

Dr. Long was from Haiphong, North Vietnam, and was very bitter about the bombing of his city by US forces. He did not like Americans. We clashed at first, but gradually became friends because of our mutual interest in orthopaedics. He was very innovative. He figured out that he could use honey to store bone graft. He would harvest bone from a donor patient and store it in honey until he could use it to fill a defect in another patient's bone. Honey has sterilizing properties and can also be used in open wounds. Dr. Long also developed carbon fiber implants that can be used to replace damaged bone. His ideas were so good that international commercial companies are now developing them.

Dr. Phung, Director of the Hospital for Traumatology and Orthopaedics (HTO) in Ho Chi Minh City, supervises many innovative Vietnamese surgeons. Dr. Vo Van Thanh, for example, worked at HTO and developed an ingenious technique for doing advanced spine surgery. Pioneering surgeons in the US and Europe required an expensive C-arm (an x-ray machine commonly used in the US that gives surgeons live images of implants and screws) in the operating room in order to accurately position metal screws into the pedicles of their patients' vertebrae. Dr. Van Thanh did the same surgery without C-arm by using a curette to accurately make the hole for the pedicle screw. He also practiced on monkeys so that he could teach himself minimally invasive techniques to correct spinal deformities like scoliosis using an arthroscope.

In 1999, Dr. Linh, also at HTO, was the first to use the SIGN Nail to lengthen a bone around the nail. This procedure transports a segment of healthy bone along the nail to fill spaces where bone has been lost or infected. The surgeon first inserts a SIGN Nail into the medullary canal of the injured extremity from top to bottom, spanning the defect. He then cuts a healthy segment of bone above the defect and spears it from the outside with threaded pins. The pins are placed perpendicular to the long axis of the bone. He attaches the ends of these pins to an external frame assembled parallel to the injured extremity. The surgeon incrementally slides the pins along the frame in turn, forcing the attached segment of bone to move over the SIGN Nail. When the process of transporting the bone segment is done properly, the patient naturally forms new bone in the space left behind by the moving segment. The innovative Vietnamese surgeons made their own external fixation devices to accomplish this procedure.

Those three phone calls in one day convinced me to shift my attention from Indonesia to Vietnam. I was fortunate to meet and work with a number of surgeons in Vietnam who inspired me with their creativity, determination, and dedication. Although I changed my focus, I can never forget the Indonesian Man in the Bed. He continues to be an inspiration for me and all SIGN Surgeons. Together our goal is to get as many patients as possible out of bed and walking again.

The key to this goal has been the SIGN Nail. It was the Vietnamese surgeons like Drs. Quang, Tuan, Long, Phung, Van Thanh, and Linh that challenged me to develop an intramedullary implant that they could use on patients who had broken legs. Once their English was good enough, they asked me to turn on a light bulb like my old mentor, Dr. Burkhalter would do. They demanded that I help them make an implant that could be inserted without an expensive fluroscope and without tools that relied on electricity. We respected the ideas that failed as well as those that were successful. I hope you will see that, like my mentors before me, we weren't afraid to act on the inspiration of an idea to improve a bad situation.

Chapter 5

Finding the Sweet Spot:
Effective Education and Appropriate Implants

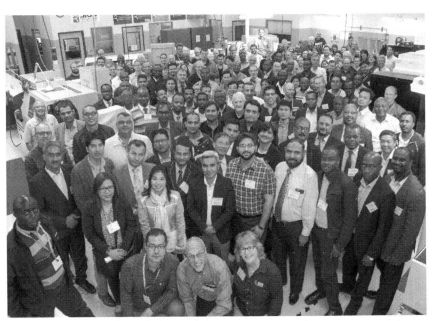

Around 150 surgeons gather each year in Richland, WA, to teach and learn from each other at the SIGN Conference.

My experience in Sumatra with the Indonesian man confined to the bed convinced me that any attempt to improve fracture care in the developing world must couple education and resources.

In Indonesia, I thought that giving lectures and operating with surgeons was sufficient. However, I learned (and other educators agree) that education is much more than giving a lecture. Just listening to words is a very inefficient way to learn something new, as the graphic below illustrates. We need to actively engage our senses, our minds, and our hands in order to really learn a new procedure.

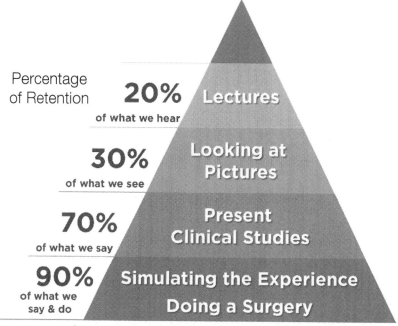

We must supplement lectures by encouraging presentation of clinical studies and donating appropriate implants to implement the education.

We only retain 20 percent of what we hear in lecture. However, we remember 70 percent of that information if we give the lecture.[2] One of the best ways to learn something is to teach it. SIGN sponsors an annual conference where surgeons from all over the world come and give talks about their experiences using SIGN Implants to help

---

2 Atesok, Kivanc, MD. "Retention of Skills After Simulations-Based Training in Orthopaedic Surgery." *Journal of the American Academy of Orthopaedic Surgeons* 24, no. 8 (August 2016). doi:10.5435/JAAOS-D-15-00440.

facilitate this model of education. We are honored that each year the keynote speaker is the president of the Orthopaedic Trauma Association.

Surgeons remember 90 percent of the information gained by performing an operation through simulations, participating in clinical studies, or doing the surgery. SIGN Surgeons, therefore, must have access to simulations using appropriate implants to implement the knowledge they hear in lectures. We have designed simulators to practice aspects of the surgery in addition to designing appropriate implants so the surgeons can implement their education and treat the poor.

Our personal biases and egos are factors that influence how well we learn. For example, a rooster crows every day at dawn. Since the sun comes up every time he crows in the morning, he is biased to believe that his crowing causes the sun to rise. A surgeon can, likewise, admire the healed bone in his patient's x-rays and believe his surgery is responsible for the good result. The surgeon, however, can be as biased as the rooster. Just as the sun does not rely on a signal from the rooster to rise, the fracture does not completely rely on the surgery to heal. There are many factors that determine fracture healing that are important. The *Fracture Healing Mind Map* on page 60 shows some of the variables that influence bone healing. Many of these are difficult to measure or control. Only the subjects on the left side can be influenced, but not controlled completely, by the surgeon.

One way to reduce the negative impact that biases have on our behavior is to record and measure our results and make that data available for review. Every SIGN Surgeon is asked to submit the radiographs of their SIGN Surgeries with reports to the SIGN Surgical Database. We record these reports, which include pre-op, post-op, and follow-up x-rays, so we can all learn together. Our original intent for the database was to verify that the SIGN Implant was capable of holding fractured bones together long enough to allow healing.

FRACTURE HEALING
MIND MAP

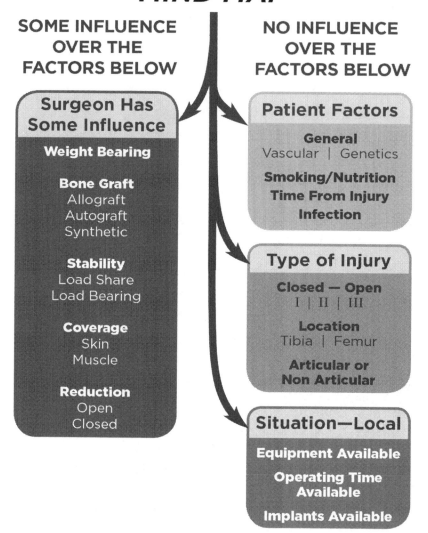

SOME INFLUENCE OVER THE FACTORS BELOW

Surgeon Has Some Influence

Weight Bearing

Bone Graft
Allograft
Autograft
Synthetic

Stability
Load Share
Load Bearing

Coverage
Skin
Muscle

Reduction
Open
Closed

NO INFLUENCE OVER THE FACTORS BELOW

Patient Factors

General
Vascular | Genetics

Smoking/Nutrition
Time From Injury
Infection

Type of Injury

Closed — Open
I | II | III

Location
Tibia | Femur

Articular or Non Articular

Situation—Local

Equipment Available

Operating Time Available

Implants Available

The surgeon must remain humble because many factors that influence healing are not under the surgeon's control.

Review of the database x-rays proved that the SIGN Nail maintains fracture stabilization. Reviews of the database also demonstrated that the infection rate is low.[3,4]

The SIGN Database continues to grow in number of x-rays submitted and results of SIGN Surgery continue to improve. We always remain humble because the follow-up x-rays show whether the fracture has healed or not. An example of an emerging pattern of healing is the use of the retrograde approach, through the knee, to stabilize fractures in the distal femur. Furthermore, we suggest that the fin nail be used for fractures in the high stress area of the femur. Screw holes in a standard interlocking nail are stress concentrators, which predispose the patient to fracture after recurrent trauma. We share this information with the surgeons.

SIGN Surgeons and I discuss difficult fractures through the comment section of the database. We continue to learn together. The increase in number of follow-up reports allows us to look at the entire fracture healing process and discuss ways to improve our results. We also document and discuss novel treatments using SIGN Implants. The follow-up reports are the report card of the orthopaedic surgeon. When I am in the United States, I review each report and send comments to the surgeons about their surgeries. When I am away, David Whitney, an orthopaedic surgeon on the SIGN Board reviews the reports and makes comments.

3   Young, Sven; Lie, Stein Atle; Hallan, Geir; Zirkle, Lewis G.; Engesæter, Lars B.; and Havelin, Leif I. "Risk factors for infection after 46,113 intramedullary nail operations in low- and middle-income countries." World Journal of Surgery 37, no. 2 (October 02, 2012): 349-55. doi:10.1007/s00268-012-1817-4.

4   Young, Sven; Lie, Stein Atle; Hallan, Geir; Zirkle, Lewis G.; Engesæter, Lars B.; and Havelin, Leif I. "Low infection rates after 34,361 intramedullary nail operations in 55 low- and middle-income countries." Acta Orthopaedica 82, no. 6 (December 09, 2011): 737-43. doi:10.3109/17453674.2011.636680.

My Indonesian experience taught me that in order to equip local surgeons to treat broken limbs, we had to provide both the knowledge and the resources for treating fractures. It was not until I had been called back to Vietnam, however, that I began to appreciate what the appropriate resources were and how they should be provided to the surgeons who could use them. The emphasis here is on the word "appropriate" because conditions are different for surgery in developing countries. Combining effective education with the right implants brought SIGN to a "sweet spot" conducive for promoting the equality of fracture care.

The sweet spot is a balance between two opposing forces such as work and play or nourishment and gluttony. Fracture healing involves sweet spots. Orthopaedic surgeons have constantly sought a balance between doing procedures to promote fracture union versus interfering with the bone's natural capacity to heal. Ancient Egyptians, for example, used bamboo splints and plaster to reduce suffering in their patients by stabilizing fractures and decreasing pain. In modern times, surgeons incise the soft tissues next to the broken bone and implant metal devices to hold the fracture pieces together. This approach allows patients to move their injured limbs right away and speeds return to a normal life. Sometimes, however, the incisions made to place the implants also allow bacteria to get into the wound, causing infection that could result in the patient's death. Finding the sweet spot in treating fractures involves deciding whether to use a splint or an implant. In other words, surgeons must determine which fractures need surgical intervention and how much intervention is required. Finding the sweet spot for SIGN involves designing implants that can be used in austere environments and then evaluating the results of surgery using these implants. In order to come up with a device that surgeons could use anywhere in the world, we stood on the shoulders of giants in the history of orthopaedic surgery.

Dr. Gerhard Küntscher was one of these giants. In his book, *The Marrow Nailing Method*, published in 1947, Professor Dr. Küntscher describes his journey innovating and inventing what he called the "marrow nail." Küntscher invented a stainless steel nail designed to go down the medullary canal of the femur to immobilize the fracture. He studied the location of the fracture and possible complications, such as infection. He attempted to find his own "sweet spot" between surgical and nonsurgical treatment. This quest to provide optimal fracture treatment continues. Küntscher described the interlocking process by placing a screw through both sides of the bone canal and through the slot in the nail after it is placed into the canal. This controlled rotation and slipping of the fracture. This technique of "locking" the nail in the bone was developed years after his publication.

Among Küntscher's early patients were World War II American pilots and crews who broke their femurs when the Germans shot down their planes. These patients surprised their American doctors when they returned after the war walking on their healed femur fractures. The US physicians were even more shocked when the x-rays of these war heroes revealed a steel rod inside the healed femur. American and European surgeons took some time to recognize the value of Küntscher's work before they developed ways to place the interlocking screws as described by Küntscher. Many people helped modify his marrow nail into today's intramedullary nail with interlocking screws. The locked intramedullary nail became the contemporary treatment of choice for fractures of the long bones of the legs and arms. The addition of the interlocking screw to the nail provided more stability for the fracture and, therefore, expanded the indications for its use.

The modern version of Küntscher's nail is considered the best choice for an implant to help patients avoid the outcome of the Indonesian man in the bed. This system was shown to provide the best stabilization for femur and tibia fractures at the time. But we had to consider the conditions in operating rooms of SIGN Surgeons. There are power surges in many operating rooms in developing countries. This means power equipment such as power reamers and x-ray imaging in the operating room cannot be used. We looked for other ways to accomplish reaming and placing the interlocking screws to stabilize the fracture without using power equipment.

Our early efforts took place in garages back home in Richland, WA. My Vietnamese colleagues and I wanted to devise a system equivalent to those used in United States. Through trial and error, we began to design the first SIGN Nail. Steve Critchlow, Dan Wodrich, and Chris Smith all contributed. We used PVC pipe, cow bones from the local butcher, and steel rods with holes drilled in their ends to accommodate the interlocking screws. Randy Huebner, founder and president of Acumed, a medical implant company in Portland, OR, heard about our attempts and visited our initial SIGN Workshop to see what we were doing. He was very patient and tactful. Randy supported my vision of a useful implant, but pointed out the limitations of my early ideas.

A major consideration was that we did not have any machines to manufacture the nails, screws, and instruments needed for the implant. I thought we could purchase hand-milling machines capable of producing the nails. We could then ship these machines with steel rods needed to manufacture the nails to Vietnam, where the surgeons could make their own implants and use them to treat patients with fractures. In retrospect, this was a bad idea. I'm sure Randy knew it would not work, but he waited for me to discover it for myself. It took me eight hours to make two nails using the hand-milling machines. This was far too much production time per nail to hope to supply enough implants for the thousands of patients who needed them in Vietnam.

Our early nail designs were not only limited by production difficulties; we had not yet discovered a technique to place the interlocking screws through the bone and slot of the nail without real-time imaging or C-arm—the method used in the United States and Europe. Real-time x-rays in the operating room allow the surgeon to align the fracture fragments, create an entry hole for the implant, as well as guide an interlocking screw across the bone through a slot in the nail. These machines are not affordable and cannot be used if there are power surges. We needed to devise another way to reliably place the interlocking screws. How could we shoot the bullseye through the slot of the nail when it was buried inside the bone canal and all we could see was our incision down to the bone?

Part of the solution was a target arm that could be placed on the outside of the limb and temporarily attached to the implant. This tool could line up a drill guide on the outside of the bone with the nail hole inside the medullary canal. This technique was very useful for placing the screw in the holes nearest the proximal end of the nail. Using this device and a small incision through the overlying soft tissues, the surgeon could hit the bullseye of the hole in the implanted nail by drilling through one side of the bone, across the hole in the nail, and out the other side of the bone. Once the bone pieces are secured this way, they cannot slide or rotate around the nail. The stability created by locking each end of the broken bone to the nail allows for early weight bearing and fracture healing. (See Appendix for details and figures of SIGN Surgery.)

As I mentioned, Randy Huebner endorsed the idea of using implants to treat the poor. He authorized Acumed to manufacture the first SIGN Nails and Target Arm. Acumed had developed a target arm for their own nail used to stabilize humerus (arm) fractures. This target arm guided the insertion of the screws placed through the nail nearest the shoulder. It worked very well and Acumed used the same principle to guide the screws into the near end of the SIGN Nail. After Acumed completed this first version of the SIGN Instruments and

Implants, I carried them to Vietnam in 2000. At that time, almost all the people in Vietnam were poor. I realized, even with a target arm instead of a fluoroscope, SIGN Implants would be complicated to manufacture, and they needed to be donated to the poor.

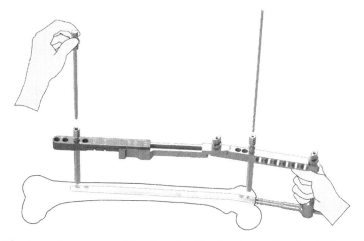

The target arm provides longitudinal orientation in finding slots in the nail.

The Vietnamese surgeons were not only receptive to the first SIGN Nail; they were enthusiastic and innovative. The initial design, like the Acumed nail, used the target arm to guide screw placement into the proximal end of the fracture. The proximal end is nearest the bone entrance while the distal end is farthest from the bone entrance. We soon discovered that placing interlocking screws through the distal end using only a target arm was very difficult. Sometimes the target arm or the position of the two fracture fragments shifted after the hole in the cortex was drilled. Sometimes the nail bent during insertion, making placement of the distal interlocking screw difficult and sometimes impossible. We looked for ways to reliably place the distal interlocking screw.

The Vietnamese surgeons and I had many discussions as we exchanged ideas for placing the distal interlocking screws.

Perhaps, they suggested, we could see the distal hole in the nail once it was inside the canal of the bone by shining a bright light through it. We could then point our drill at the bright spot on the outside of the bone and drill through the target. To test this idea, we drilled a hole in the end of a Küntscher nail, implanted the nail in a cadaver bone, put a bright light on a stick, and ran the light down the center of the nail. Unfortunately, it didn't shine through the bone and soft tissues and we couldn't discern where the nail's distal hole was located.

I had noticed that the Vietnamese surgeons had a refined sense of touch. They trained their fingers to provide information about the fracture that most orthopaedic surgeons glean with their eyes. This was because the Vietnamese doctors didn't have access to the real-time imaging in the operating room. They would make a small incision over the fracture site and adroitly manipulate the fragments into alignment with their fingers. It occurred to me that this tactile skill could be used to locate the distal hole in the nail and allow accurate screw placement. This tactile skill is stimulated by vibrations at the end of the instrument which indicate the location of the instrument as well as irregularities such as the slot in the nail.

We developed instruments called slot finders to utilize tactile sense in finding the slot in the nail. We continue to improve the slot finders and study the location of the slots in the nail after the nail is inserted into the bone canal. We must not only discover these things for ourselves, but we must communicate them to SIGN Surgeons. We made an animated video showing what happens inside the canal as the nail is introduced. I had wondered many times what was happening as the nail was placed down the bone canal. For me, making these animated videos was like a blind person regaining their sight. I had wondered for many years what was happening inside the canal when I had difficulty finding the slot in the nail to place the distal interlocking screw. Randy made the first SIGN Simulator using wood and plastic.

Further illumination came when we developed simulators using clear plexiglas tubes to simulate the bone with the nail. We drilled holes in the plexiglas and used slot finders to simulate finding the slot in the hole. Throughout this process, I was reminded of Einstein's statement "Knowledge is limited. Imagination encircles the world."[5] In 2013, The United States Patent and Trademark Office recognized our designs and innovations by awarding SIGN their Patents for Humanity Award for our implants and instruments.

Our next challenge was manufacturing the instruments and implants. Acumed and Randy gave us our first machines to manufacture SIGN Implants and Instruments in 1999. Within three months after installing the machines in a workshop in Richland, we found people that had the skills we needed to run the machines and manufacture orthopaedic implants. These people included Dule Mehic, who escaped from the Bosnian War. He initially fled from Bosnia to Germany and then came to the United States. He had some difficulty with the English language, but he obviously knew how to program and run milling machines. He helped get our first machines operating and now is engaged with designing instruments to be manufactured on these machines.

Richard Grizzell also showed up for a tour of SIGN. He taught a machinist course in Walla Walla, WA. He was injured in an auto accident and is an incomplete paraplegic. After his tour of our original factory, he agreed to train our machinists how to program and operate a newly acquired machine and soon joined our staff. His inability to walk does not handicap his productivity. He can lock his knees to stand, and I've seen him up on ladders while working at SIGN. He became the leader of manufacturing at SIGN.

Sean Bradley came to work for SIGN just out of machinist school in nearby Yakima, WA. His school had taught him how to operate

---

5   Barna, Mark. "The Heroes of Science." *Discover Magazine, May 2017, 37.*

milling machines, but we quickly realized that our machines needed additional programming. He took my personal computer home and used it to teach himself how to program the machines to do what we needed.

Thanks to Dule, Richard, Sean, and many others, SIGN now has very talented manufacturing and engineering departments. The story of engineering at SIGN is discussed further in *A Leg to Stand On* by Dr. Michelle Foltz, a book about the early days of SIGN. It is well done and I recommend it. Michelle traveled to developing countries so she could observe the value of SIGN as a surgeon and an author.

Jeanne Dillner was a consultant to the International Atomic Energy Agency in Vienna when she first visited SIGN in 1999. Although trained as a certified public accountant, Jeanne immediately understood the philosophy of SIGN. I asked her how we could measure our success, and she said, "by the number of patients we treat." I soon asked her to become the Chief Executive Officer of SIGN. She understands the scope of SIGN because she accompanies me on trips to developing countries. Jeanne coordinates the activities of all departments and nearly 40 employees. Her leadership has been crucial to our continuing success.

The development of slot finders and an external target arm allowed SIGN to manufacture an implant with all the advantages of the modern version of Küntscher's nail (with interlocking screws), which was usable in the austere operating environment of Vietnam.

In addition to those I've highlighted here, many more people have contributed to the continuing success of SIGN. Surgeons around the world, staff at our headquarters, and generous supporters push us to fulfill our ambition of creating equality of fracture care throughout the world. We continue to improve by incremental changes.

Chapter 6

Diversity Promotes Innovation

The first SIGN Nail was initially made for Vietnamese tibias. The nail was manufactured with very little curve to match the straight canal of the tibial bone. We focused on tibia fractures because they were so common in Vietnam and a high number of complications occur in these injuries. Unlike other long bones in the body, the tibia doesn't have a muscle and soft tissue covering, so the tibia is often exposed to contamination when it is fractured. This can lead to infection and amputation of the lower leg if not treated properly.

My Vietnamese associates began expanding the use of the SIGN Nail as soon as I introduced it to them. In 2000, an 18-year-old girl with a fracture of both her tibia and femur was admitted to Cho Ray Hospital in Ho Chi Minh City. We first stabilized her tibia using the SIGN Nail in the standard fashion. Since the girl could not afford a curved nail designed for the femur, we placed another SIGN Nail into her femur through her knee, using the same incision we made for her tibia. At the time, we were not aware of other surgeons who had used this approach to stabilize a fractured thighbone. Later we found that other trauma surgeons in Europe and the US were beginning to use this technique. After I returned home, the surgeon sent me a picture of the girl standing on her fractured leg six weeks after her surgery. I was elated to see the result and was encouraged that the SIGN Nail could be used for both tibia and femur fractures when both bones are broken in the same leg from a motorcycle accident.

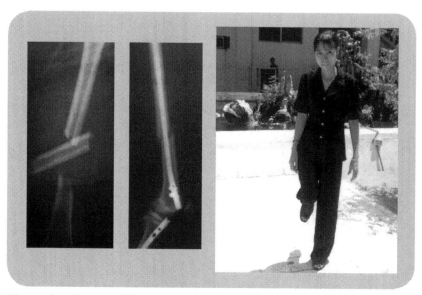

Six weeks after receiving two SIGN Implants to stabilize her femur and tibia, this young woman was able to stand and walk on her injured leg.

Two weeks later, I received a letter from Dr. Han Khoi Quang with an x-ray showing the straight SIGN Nail implanted to treat another Vietnamese femur fracture. This time Dr. Quang inserted the nail from the hip side of the bone, rather than introducing the implant through the knee. Dr. Quang astutely informed me that the SIGN Nail worked very well when used this way for femur fractures. We did not have to change the design of our tibial nail to fit the curved femur. He suggested that the surgeon allow the slight proximal bend in our nail (which we manufactured to allow ease of placement in the tibia) to rotate as it was inserted across the helical configuration of the proximal femur. Our nail could rotate inside the femur and follow the bony contour because it wasn't enlarged at its end to hold a large diameter locking screw like most femoral intramedullary implants. Dr. Quang's technique demonstrated that our straight tibial nail could be used and locked for either left or right femurs. SIGN didn't need to develop and manufacture a different nail to use for femur fractures.

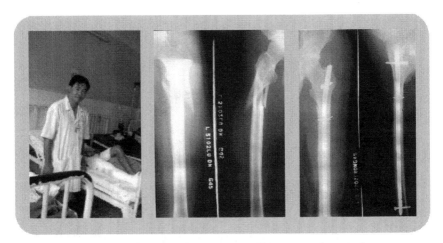

Dr. Quang pioneered using the SIGN Nail to treat femur fractures, as seen in these x-ray images.

The application of new SIGN Techniques as well as new implants expanded as the group of dedicated surgeons, the SIGN Family, grew. Once we began publishing our results, trauma surgeons from all over the world began to request our free implants. Soon after I brought the SIGN Nail to India, Dr. Nicholas Antao of Mumbai placed the first SIGN Nail into a fractured humerus. A short time later, Professor Thit Lwin of Myanmar used a SIGN Nail to fuse an arthritic ankle joint by inserting the nail through the foot.

Dr. Faruque Quasem heard about SIGN and asked us to start a program in his hospital in Dhaka, Bangladesh. I brought him a set of our SIGN Nails, the Target Arm, slot finders, and hand reamers that we had developed to treat the patients in Vietnam. We had decided to use hand reamers to enlarge the canal of the bone for placement of the nail because frequent power surges or lack of electricity in developing countries prevented the use of power reaming. The decision to avoid power tools for implanting the nail proved fortunate in several ways in Bangladesh. They had no electricity in many of their operating rooms, so Faruque and I operated by the light of the window.

More importantly, using the hand reamers led to the development of a new SIGN Implant, the Fin Nail.

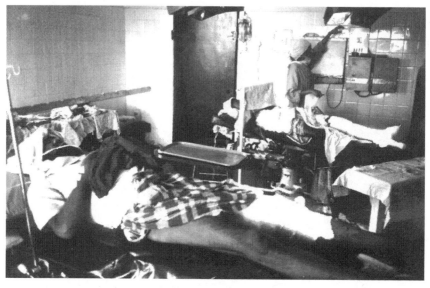

The 1st SIGN Surgery in Bangladesh was done by the light of the window without C-arm or power instruments.

The bone of the Bangladeshi patients was much harder than bones of people in Vietnam. Our hand drills, which worked so well in Vietnam, often skived off the outside of the hard bone in Bangladesh, making placement of the interlocking screws agonizingly difficult. The hand reamers, which passed easily through Vietnamese medullary canals, were difficult to pass through the canals of the Bangladeshi bone.

Despite our struggles with the instruments, we decided to do one more surgery before I had to leave for my flight home. During this last case, the hand reamer became stuck in the canal of the femur. It would not advance and I had a great deal of trouble removing it. We completed the case just in time for me to catch my plane. I left Bangladesh very frustrated from the experience.

A few weeks later, I was riding my bicycle home from the office when a light bulb turned on over my head. We could get around the problems of skiving hand drills by eliminating the need for the distal interlocking screws. The jammed reamers provided inspiration for this innovation. We could place the reamer tip config-uration at the distal end of the nail. There would be no need to place a screw through the end of the nail because the flutes would anchor it inside the bony canal, just as the reamer stuck in the femur in Bangladesh.

We subsequently designed and manufactured the Fin Nail. The Fin Nail has proven very effective for femoral fractures. In order to make room for flutes at the end of the nail, hand reaming must enlarge the canal of the bone. In the process of accommodating for the larger end of the Fin Nail, hand reaming also straightens the curved shape of the canal. This allows the Fin Nail to pass easily into the femur. It also provides three major points of support of the bony fragments around the nail—at its midpoint and its two ends. This triangular buttressing of the bone holds the broken pieces of the femur firmly together and pushes the fin against the side of the canal.

The SIGN Hand Reamers provide bone from the canal during reaming, which can be used to accelerate fracture healing. We are also experimenting with mechanical stimulation of stem cells in cortical bone from the fracture site using our bone mill, which will also accelerate fracture healing.

Dr. Sven Young, from Norway, has published two articles com-paring infection rates in surgeries where the fracture site was opened and stabilized with a SIGN Nail compared to surgeries that don't open the fracture site, using conventional intramedullary implants. He found no difference in the infection rates, demonstrating that our technique of opening the fracture and operating without a C-arm is effective and safe.[6,7]

Joel Gillard (an engineer formerly employed by Acumed and who now works for SIGN) and Randy Huebner modified the design of the hand reamers so they would harvest more marrow. Joel also worked with Randy's son, Kyle, to develop a sharpener for these reamers.

Surgeons around the world contribute to the effectiveness of the SIGN System. Surgeons from the Philippines, for example, presented a new idea at a SIGN Conference. They minimized the opening over the fracture site to a size that allowed them to insert only one finger in order to guide the reamers and the nail. They explained that this technique resulted in less post-operative pain and required less bone grafting when the soft tissue around the fracture was minimally disturbed. Duane Anderson, a SIGN Surgeon in Ethiopia, has designed a traction apparatus to hold the fracture out to length while awaiting surgery. He employs a disabled man to supervise the design and manufacture of these traction devices as well as operating room tables and wheelchairs. Both the idea of the Philippine finger and the constant traction benefit the patient by reducing operating time and achieving better results.

Many fractures, unfortunately, cannot be manipulated with only a finger. Many patients in the developing world cannot get to a hospital until weeks after they suffer a broken bone. By this time the broken bone is often shortened, deformed, and beginning to knit together

---

6   Young, Sven; Lie, Stein Atle; Hallan, Geir; Zirkle, Lewis G.; Engesæter, Lars B.; and Havelin, Leif I. "Risk factors for infection after 46,113 intramedullary nail operations in low- and middle-income countries." World Journal of Surgery 37, no. 2 (October 02, 2012): 349-55. doi:10.1007/s00268-012-1817-4.

7   Young, Sven; Lie, Stein Atle; Hallan, Geir; Zirkle, Lewis G.; Engesæter, Lars B.; and Havelin, Leif I. "Low infection rates after 34,361 intramedullary nail operations in 55 low- and middle-income countries." Acta Orthopaedica 82, no. 6 (December 09, 2011): 737-43. doi:10. 3109/17453674.2011.636680.

in poor position. Pulling these partially healed pieces apart in order to reduce the fracture can be difficult and uses precious operating room time. The distractor we designed in response to the overriding fractures after the Pakistan earthquake has been improved upon and is now sold by Innomed.

Fusing Joints

We have discovered that the SIGN Nail can fuse joints that are painfully worn out by arthritis. In the US and Europe these patients are treated with total knee and total hip replacements. Poor people in the developing world cannot afford sophisticated artificial joint replacements. The alternative treatment is to fuse the joint. I mentioned how a SIGN Surgeon in Myanmar fused an arthritic ankle with our nail. SIGN Surgeons around the world have now used this technique, called retrocalcaneal fusion, in over 150 surgeries.

At Eldoret Hospital in Kenya, a woman was admitted with a femur fracture. She complained more from the pain in her chronically arthritic knee than she did from her recently broken femur. She asked us to address the painful worn out joint as well as fix her broken thighbone. After a long night of discussing the options with Kenyan surgeons and me, Dr. Kibor Lelei decided to use one SIGN Nail from the hip down to stabilize her fractured femur and use another nail to fuse her knee. He cut out the arthritic portions of her knee joint and held the prepared surfaces solidly together with the SIGN Nail. I saw this woman the morning after surgery. She had to share a bed with another woman because there were not enough hospital beds for all the patients. When she recognized us, however, she had a big smile on her face because her knee pain was already less.

Duane Anderson, Bob Greene, and other surgeons in Ethiopia have also used the SIGN Nail to not only treat acute fractures but also to correct deformities that have resulted from fractures that have healed in malalignment. Duane was asked to help a young girl whose knees were fixed in a 90-degree backward position from previous fractures. She had to walk backwards on her hands and feet. Duane and Bob released the abnormal bend in the girl's knees and held the damaged joints straight by fusing her knees with a SIGN Nail. Her knees were now held with a slight bend that allowed her to walk normally. This correction gave her a completely new outlook on life and tremendous joy as she now truly had a future.

Bone Loss

Another condition that can result in deformity after a fracture is bone loss. A defect can be caused initially when the energy of the injury is great enough to destroy sections of the bone or it can result from an infection or from a congenital abnormality. As I previously mentioned, Vietnamese SIGN Surgeons pioneered the technique of using the SIGN Nail in transporting bone to fill a defect. Dr. Rich Gellman and Dr. John Herzenberg are world-renowned authorities on correcting limb deformities. They now teach new SIGN Surgeons how to use this "bone lengthening" technique at the annual SIGN Conference.

We wondered how well the SIGN Nail would hold fracture fragments in place until healing. This question was studied using an on-screen protractor developed by Sasha Carson, Sam Si-Hyeong Park, David A. Simon, and Robert Feibel who showed that the stability of the fracture stabilized by the SIGN Nail was equivalent to other IM nails[8]. Andrew Tice, Sasha Carsen, and others used a similar method to study the stability of the Fin Nail and found that it was as stable as a standard SIGN Nail, except where the bone was fractured in many pieces.

---

8   Carsen, Sasha; Park, Sam Si-Hyeong; Simon, David A.; and Feibel, Robert J. "Treatment With the SIGN Nail in Closed Diaphyseal Femur Fractures Results in Acceptable Radiographic Alignment." Clinical Orthopaedics and Related Research® 473, no. 7 (July 17, 2015): 2394-401. doi:10.1007/s11999-015-4290-1.

Blast and Gunshot Injuries

SIGN Fracture Care International's goal is to provide the education and equipment necessary to treat the entire injury. An open fracture in which the bone is exposed because the muscles and skin are damaged is a very severe injury. Open fractures are more common in developing countries. One of the most devastating types of open fractures occurs as a result of high velocity gunshot wounds and explosions.

SIGN Surgeons in Afghanistan like Dr. Ismail Wardak and his colleagues in Pakistan have placed SIGN Nails in open fractures caused by gunshot wounds and blast injuries, with good results. These surgeons have so many wounded patients and so little available operating room time that they have implanted the nails in these mangled limbs sooner than reported elsewhere in the orthopaedic literature. They have also become quite efficient using our nail. Dr. Wardak presented a video showing him implanting a SIGN Nail in a fractured tibia in four minutes! Dr. Wardak and his associates have not only demonstrated fast surgeries, their results with immediate nailing of fractures from gunshots and blasts show up on the SIGN Database with quicker healing times and lower rates of infection than would be expected. We don't encourage speed in surgery, but it is important to be efficient because operating room time is at a premium in developing countries.

I was so intrigued by results treating fractures from bullets and bombs that I consulted Jim Green, a retired engineer from Synthes, one of the world's leading orthopaedic implant manufacturers, to review these results and try to explain them. Jim theorized that these war-time fractures sustain so much force that stem cells, normally trapped in the overlying cortical bone, are released when the bone is shattered from an explosion or high velocity bullet. These cells, in turn, provide a powerful stimulus to bone healing. He explained that these results correlate with laboratory studies that have unveiled these potent cells hidden in the recesses of cortical bone. Jim's explanation helped turn on another SIGN "light bulb": If a blast injury can unleash this healing force, maybe we can use these cells to help the bone heal in a more typical fracture. SIGN is now manufacturing a bone mill to grind up some of the cortical bone at the fracture site and then implant it so that the previously trapped stem cells released from the milling process can accelerate union of the broken bone.

Soft Tissue Defects

Correcting soft-tissue defects is as important as stabilizing the fracture. I was giving grand rounds in 2005 at Duke University School of Medicine and met Dr. Scott Levin. Dr. Levin is a world-famous surgeon who is now Chief of Orthopaedic and Plastic Surgery at the University of Pennsylvania. He recently performed the world's first successful bilateral hand transplantation. In 2005, he showed me his lab at Duke and suggested that he could give a course to SIGN Surgeons about optimal management of soft tissue injuries associated with open fractures. This involves transferring tissues over the bone to replace the damaged tissues. I chose six promising young surgeons from all over the world who traveled to Duke University in order to learn soft-tissue coverage from Dr. Levin. These surgeons now contribute to orthopaedic knowledge not only in their country but in the world. Dr. Bhaskar Pant was an orthopaedic resident in the Philippines at the time of this first soft tissue management course. He now works in Nepal. Since completing Dr. Levin's course, Dr. Bhaskar has performed three hand re-implantations. This illustrates how SIGN educational resources can be taken home by surgeons to benefit patients in their own countries.

Dr. Randy Sherman, chief of the Division of Plastic Surgery at Cedars-Sinai Medical Center in Los Angeles, CA, has helped us expand the training first offered by Dr. Levin. For the next six years, Randy sponsored the SIGN Flap Course at the University of Southern California School of Medicine. The course then moved to San Francisco under the leadership of the Institute for Global Orthopaedics and Traumatology (IGOT) and the University of San Francisco. Their efforts have increased the number of SIGN Surgeons who can attend the course each year. The IGOT staff has renamed their course the Surgical Management and Reconstructive Training Course (SMART Course), and it is attended by new SIGN Surgeons each year.

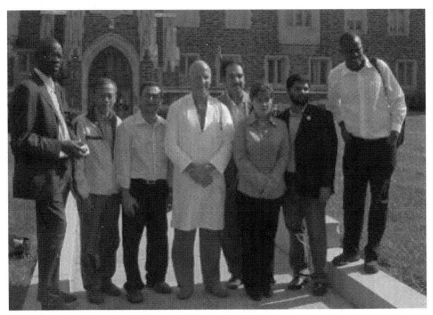

Dr. Scott Levin (white coat, center) with a group of SIGN Surgeons attending the SIGN Flap Course.

Negative pressure wound therapy is a method of treating soft tissue injuries. This technique applies a constant negative pressure to the injury in order to promote healing and decrease infection. This is an effective but expensive process in the United States. SIGN Surgeons have made the treatment affordable in their own countries by using cheap aquarium pumps to provide the negative pressure. The results are good. Dr. Kim Jingco from the Philippines developed a website where he discussed new techniques to use negative pressure wound therapy. Other organizations such as COAN and MIT are working on similar low-cost models.

Infections

Infection is a problem in open fractures, and SIGN Surgeons have studied different methods to decrease the possibility of infection. Some surgeons use bleach and tap water to cleanse the wound, while others put powdered antibiotic in the wound. Sometimes antibiotic is added to methyl methacrylate cement and placed in the wound to give a constant high dose of antibiotic. Our growing network of SIGN Surgeons around the world is studying different methods of preventing infection in hopes to find the optimal treatment.

By means of sharing our experiences using the database and through our organized conferences, SIGN Surgeons are learning to reduce complications of open fractures by cleaning the wound and stabilizing the broken bone with SIGN Implants. Stability is an important aspect of preventing infection of the bone, and we are now studying the optimal timing for placing the nail. SIGN Surgeons do not have the operating room time to do repeated cleansing of wounds, and they are finding that placing the nail and closing the wound earlier is working. The SIGN Nail is a solid nail. It has less surface area than most ordinary intramedullary implants, which are shaped like tubes. The SIGN Nail, therefore, has less surface area for bacteria to make a home in the nail and infect the bone. As we learn more about the genetics of bacteria and their ways of survival, I wonder if the approach in the future will be to strive to allow the patient back to activity by closing the wound and inserting the SIGN Nail much earlier. I don't think we can ever remove all bacteria from the wound, but perhaps we can change the environment. This approach of early soft-tissue closure and nail insertion is necessary due to lack of resources in austere environments. We must learn from this approach.

SIGN has grown into a partnership among surgeons around the world. Each member of the SIGN Family contributes to the partnership. Knowledge flows throughout the SIGN Family, and the results benefit our patients. I believe that knowledge leads to understanding and understanding leads to peace. All of us in the SIGN Family have a high regard for each other.

Early on, I was convinced that the SIGN Nail and Instruments had to be donated if we were going to really equalize fracture care in the world. Design and manufacture of implants has remained centered where it began, in Richland, WA, so we can control the cost and quality of our instruments and implants. This decision requires us to be compliant with the strict rules and regulations imposed by the United States Food and Drug Administration. We must follow the same regulations as multi-billion-dollar commercial implant companies.

The SIGN Family has grown markedly since the early days, when we were only implanting tibial nails in Vietnam. The family has expanded to include surgeons all over the world. Their creativity and needs have expanded our ability to treat fractures of all the long bones in the body, to use SIGN Nails to correct deformities, alleviate crippling arthritis, and stabilize the most severe open fractures. The family has grown to include engineers and scientists who have helped us manufacture new implants, correlate and measure our data, and teach new techniques. Finally, our family includes managers and staff who coordinate the efforts of all the family members so we can equalize fracture care. Jeanne Dillner guides this team with great skill and wisdom.

The story and the family of SIGN Fracture International grew from a simple tibial intramedullary implant. The story continues, however, with the advent of two other important orthopaedic implants.

Chapter 7

The SIGN Hip Construct and Pediatric Fracture Implants

The original reason for SIGN was to equalize treatment of the ubiquitous tibia fracture in the developing world. The efforts of creative SIGN Surgeons established that in addition to use in the tibia, the nail was effective for treating fractures in the femur and the humerus. SIGN Surgeons also demonstrated the implant could be effective treating open fractures as well as addressing limb deformities and arthritis of the knee and ankle joints.

SIGN Hip Construct

We began to contemplate whether we should design and manufacture implants to treat other fractures. This decision was influenced by an x-ray from Cambodia submitted to the SIGN Database showing treatment of a very severe hip fracture with the standard SIGN Nail. I asked the surgeon to send follow-up reports. I knew from experience that hip fractures are very different from other long bone fractures. Three months later, I received an x-ray and a video of the patient walking without a limp. This was good news, but I remembered that "one rose does not make a rose garden." I also knew that the standard SIGN Nail would not work in every hip fracture.

We were contemplating this decision of expanding to design and manufacture other implants when I was called to Pakistan to treat

85

earthquake survivors. As I looked up at the hills surrounding the hospital where we were operating, I remembered the Nelson Mandela quote, "After climbing a great hill, one only finds there are more hills to climb." I was inspired that, even amid the other great challenges we were overcoming, we also needed to climb the hill of hip fractures.

I remember visiting Myanmar in 1997 and being told that patients with broken hips were sent home to die because they could not move in their bed and developed pressure sores that became infected. Ten years later in Afghanistan, we were told that patients with hip fractures were treated by bed traction for three weeks and then sent home in a cast. It is extremely cold in Afghanistan and nobody except the US Army received electricity more than six hours per day. We didn't know which six hours. We could go to bed very warm and wake up freezing or pile on the covers and wake up very warm when the electricity came on. I imagined a person in a cast that cannot move trying to cope with this. SIGN is driven by response to patient needs, and these experiences convinced me that we should design and manufacture a system to treat hip fractures.

To be useful in hospitals in developing countries, SIGN needed to come up with an implant for hip fractures that could be placed without x-ray guidance. We had done this for the tibia so we were confident we could do it for the hip. Putting a broken hip together and holding it steady until the bone can heal required several special considerations.

Our implant had to be strong enough to treat all hip fractures as if they were unstable. Not all fractures of the femur around the hip joint are created equal. They are traditionally classified as stable and unstable based on their x-ray appearance. However, reliable x-rays are frequently unavailable in places like Myanmar and Afghanistan. Our implant, therefore, had to be appropriate for all types of hip fractures—unstable as well as the stable.

The implant had to work in different sizes of hips. There is a wide variation in the size of the bones in men and women in different countries. The system needed to be made up of different pieces that could be combined to fit in a variety of bone shapes and sizes.

Back at our headquarters in Richland, WA, we studied the different hip implants available in the United States. We reviewed the anatomy of the proximal femur and the biomechanical forces that the implant must resist in order to hold the fracture together. We wanted to use existing SIGN Implants and Instruments as much as possible in order to reduce the cost of manufacturing a new device for hip fractures.

Just like the Cambodian SIGN Surgeon, we began our process of addressing the hip fracture problem by using an existing SIGN Nail. We applied principles established by successful hip implants from the West. We added compression screws to our nail. These screws were directed from the outside of the proximal femur, skirted around the intramedullary nail, passed through the narrow neck of the femur, and extended into the dense bone inside the ball of the femoral head. Adding these screws to the nail allowed the implants to resist the twisting forces applied by the muscles around the joint that commonly pull unstable hip fractures apart. Unfortunately, there was not enough room in the femoral neck of Asian women to contain both the newly added compression screws and the old SIGN Interlocking Screws. We still needed the interlocking screw to keep the bone fragments from rotating or moving up and down around the nail. Therefore, we modified our original nail to accommodate the compression screws and provide room for the interlocking screw. This new nail, and associated implements, is called the SIGN Hip Construct (SHC).

We tested the construct (bone and implant) using a hydraulic press. We increased the pressure on a simulated bone implanted with our hip construct until they broke. These load-to-failure tests were initially very helpful, but the fracture often loses position in real life by repetitive stress when the patient walks, rather than one catastrophic episode modeled by our hydraulic press. We needed to simulate the forces of walking to really test our models with hip fractures stabilized by implants.

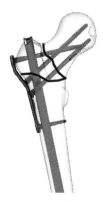

The SIGN Hip Construct was designed to treat stable and unstable fractures of the hip without using C-arm or power equipment. Results have been very good.

Justin Roth, an engineer interested in medicine, and David Shearer, a medical student from the University of Washington, visited SIGN independently during the same week. They came just as we realized we needed a different bench-testing apparatus for our hip construct. Both of them were innovative engineers interested in designing implants for use in developing countries. We discussed different methods to test the strength of our construct by simulating walking. We wanted to understand which configuration of implants provided the greatest ability to withstand repetitive stress.

Justin was working for Program for Appropriate Technology in Health (PATH) in Seattle, WA, where he obtained a grant to develop a fatigue-testing machine. Justin and Dave designed a machine that gradually put increased stress on the femoral head, as the construct moved to simulate walking. This machine has been invaluable to us for testing our hip fracture construct prototypes.

Justin graduated from medical school and is now an orthopaedic resident in Riverside, CA. He was accepted for a fellowship in pediatric orthopaedic surgery at Washington University in St. Louis, MO. Dave finished his Master of Public Health Studies at Harvard, completed his residency at the University of California of San Francisco (UCSF), and returned to the University of Washington as a trauma fellow. He is now on the staff at UCSF. Both have continued their interest in working in developing countries.

We also designed instruments to allow the surgeon to accurately place the SHC without a C-arm. In the United States, surgeons align the hip fracture fragments with a traction table in the operating room. Then they use a C-arm to visualize the fracture and the narrow portion of the femoral neck. Using the x-ray images as a guide, they drill a pin from the outside of the hip through the neck into the femoral head. This pin, in turn, forms the path for a cannulated compression screw to be inserted and hold the proximal fragments together. The guide pin is withdrawn, leaving the compression screw in place. Since our surgeons would not have real-time x-rays to see the femoral neck while they drilled a path for the compression screws, we developed a hand-held pilot instrument to provide tactile sense to the surgeon. The pilot allows the surgeon to make sure he tunnels through (and not outside) the narrow passageway of the femoral neck into hard bone under the femoral head while making an accurate track for the compression screw to follow.

We designed our compression screws with solid, rather than cannulated, shafts because our system did not rely on guide pins to position the screws. The solid shaft made our screws stronger than a similar sized hollow screw. We placed threads at both ends of the screw so they would compress the fracture fragments together, but machined them with a smooth shaft in the middle that would allow the bone pieces to collapse along the line of the screw.

There is a sweet spot in treating hip fractures that balances allowing the bone fragments to collapse enough so the pieces come together to aid healing and preventing the fragments from collapsing into an abnormal position. If the hip heals in a poor position, walking will be difficult and painful. The forces on a malunited hip can also cause it to wear out or become arthritic. Our compression screws, therefore, had to be designed to allow the broken pieces to come together while still holding the pieces firmly enough to prevent too much displacement.

After we received FDA clearance to use the SHC in November 2008, I took the implant to Afghanistan and discovered that placement of the SIGN Hip Construct requires more surgical skill than the standard SIGN Nail. SIGN Surgeons have shown great skill in using this implant. This new SIGN Implant is providing a way for surgeons to equalize treatment of hip fractures so poor people would not have to suffer in bed or body casts.

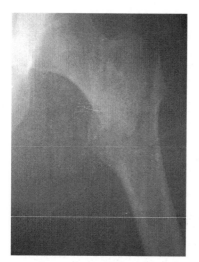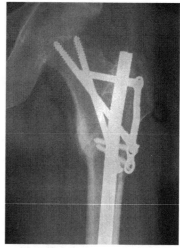

Hip fracture treated with the SIGN Hip Construct.

The design and manufacture of the SHC has improved by incremental steps. Many hip fractures extend through the lateral wall of the greater trochanter and the proximal femur. To address this, we designed a low profile, spiral plate that is held to the lateral wall of the trochanter with the proximal interlocking screw and fixed to the shaft with distal screws. The design of this plate was inspired by the helical construction of the Antoni Gaudi's Sagrada Familia in Barcelona, Spain. The helical pattern of the church's spires seemed to me an ideal shape to resist the torsional and rotational forces that can pull apart many hip fractures.

The addition of this plate to the nail not only made the construct more resistant to torsion, but also allowed the SHC to be used for treating malunited hip fractures and hip arthritis. Many patients with fractured hips who develop arthritis of the joint cannot afford artificial replacements, so we have used our compression screws and the helical plate to stabilize a corrective osteotomy. An osteotomy is an operation whereby a bone is cut to shorten, lengthen, or change its alignment.

Ariane is a 12-year-old girl with a slow growing tumor that deformed her left hip. I met her when visiting SIGN Surgeons at the Southern Philippines Medical Center in 2015. Her deformity was painful and made walking difficult. Each morning staff, residents, and tumor surgeon Dr. Rex Penaranda would visit Ariane and her father on rounds in the hospital. Ariane's father was very apprehensive of any treatment even though his daughter was becoming crippled by her tumor. "This is our only child," he told us, trying to hold back his emotions. After three mornings of discussions, planning, drawing proposed bone cuts on x-rays, and modeling the final osteotomy in three dimensions with Play-Doh, Dr. Penaranda and his associates were ready to operate. We removed Ariane's tumor, cutting the bone around her hip so it could be reassembled into a functional limb.

We stabilized the remaining healthy bone with some of the implants of the SIGN Hip Construct. The SIGN Surgeons were able to use the SHC Implants to reconstruct her proximal femur and allow her father's only child to walk again. We hope to apply corrective osteotomies like those used on Ariane's femur to change the forces on malunited and arthritic hips and allow patients to walk with less pain without having to use an expensive hip replacement.

Pediatric Fracture Implants

The SHC expanded the quiver of SIGN Implants, but adult hip fractures were not the only unsolved fracture facing our surgeons. We polled SIGN Surgeons to tell us their greatest need for implants. They stated that the number of pediatric femoral fractures were increasing faster than the number of adult femur fractures. A decrease in poverty in the developing world allowed more families to afford a motorcycle. While in the US, minivans and SUVs were used to cart children to school and soccer practice, the motorcycle was becoming the popular way to transport kids in the developing world. As more motorcycles are sold, there are more accidents and, consequently, more children are breaking their femurs.

Just like hip fractures, pediatric femur fractures were treated with a combination of bed rest, traction, and body casts. This treatment regimen, however, was using up precious hospital beds needed for more severely injured patients. It often hindered the child's ability to continue their education, imposed additional burdens on parents to tend to their hospitalized offspring, and frequently resulted in legs that were healed but shortened or deformed from the fracture. We set out to design an intramedullary implant that would address the special demands of a child's bone.

A child's femur differs from an adult in several ways. First, it is smaller in length and diameter, and often has a greater degree of curvature or anterior bow. Second, it is growing. The sources of longitudinal growth of the bone come from expanding cartilaginous caps called the epiphyses, located at both ends of the femur. The dividing cells of the epiphysis are converted to bone in a disc shaped area of its lower portion, referred to as the growth plate or physeal plate. Disruption of the physeal plate can prevent the bone from growing or deform it. Finally, pediatric bone heals much faster than adult bone. A child's bone is covered with a thick periosteal sleeve that rapidly makes new bone to replace the disrupted underlying cortex. We designed the pediatric femoral nail to allow flexibility as the nail is passed down the bowed canal in order to prevent perforation of the shaft. We discovered that an implant with a four-millimeter diameter was the largest that would allow bending of the nail during insertion.

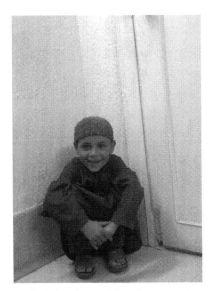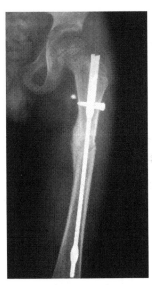

Pediatric Fin Nail has been very successful in treating pediatric femoral fractures.

Since children heal much faster than adults, we decided to use the fin concept to take the place of the interlocking screws. Interlocking screws would likely be covered over by periosteal new bone and make nail removal difficult in the child. The fin makes insertion much quicker and eases removal of the nail because the bone canal enlarges during growth. Children's fractures often heal within three to four months, so the surgeon can remove the nail with ease.

SIGN Surgeons are pleased with the results of using the pediatric femoral nail. It wasn't long before they expanded our recommended indications for using the SIGN Pediatric Nail, just as they did with the standard SIGN Nail. The first expanded indication was to place the nail in children much younger than 14 years old. I asked for follow-up reports when the patients had finished growth. So far we have detected very little growth disturbances in these younger patients.

The femoral canals of children throughout the world vary in size. In some countries, the canal was much larger, and therefore a nail with a four-millimeter diameter was too small. In response, we manufactured a pediatric nail with a six-millimeter diameter. Pediatric canals in some parts of the world were large enough for our eight-millimeter regular SIGN Fin Nails to be used. We followed all these changes in the reports submitted to the SIGN Database and found that the children healed very rapidly and did not lose reduction.

The next change noted was the use of the SIGN Pediatric Nail in fractures more distally (toward the knee). I was frankly surprised that the nail supplied enough stabilization for these fractures to heal. However, there is a limit to how far distal the SIGN Pediatric Nail would immobilize a fracture. Placing the nail just above the knee has a high complication rate because the physeal plate is located there. Fractures in this area are difficult to immobilize by placing the nail through the top of the femur. These fractures are difficult to treat using any implant.

One day, while walking down a street in Addis Ababa, Ethiopia, I was contemplating the best way to treat pediatric fractures located near the knee. Some surgeons use flexible nails, but flexible nails do not control rotation as well. Sometimes plates are used, but they are often difficult to remove and do not provide adequate immobilization.

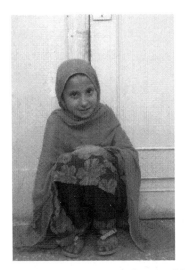 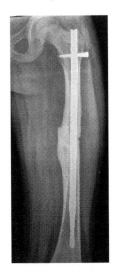

Femoral canals around the world vary in size. This seven-year-old girl was treated with a standard SIGN Fin Nail.

I saw a herd of sheep walking to market. It occurred to me that sheep might provide a way to test a novel approach for treating human pediatric fractures near the knee. The biggest challenge to treating the femur when it was broken near the knee was securing the fracture fragments without damaging the growth plate of the distal femur.

A four-month-old sheep's potential for growth is equivalent to that of a 12-year-old human. Dr. Biruk Wamisho and Dr. Woubalem Zewde, orthopaedic surgeons in Ethiopia, were our hosts during this visit, and we discussed our idea with them. Dr. Biruk knew a German veterinarian. He purchased a pair of four-month-old sheep and arranged a surgical time with the veterinarian. After we finished our SIGN Surgery on humans, we proceeded to the veterinarian's operating room.

The veterinarian was very specific about his surgical technique. We followed his guidelines for animal surgery. We placed an intramedullary rod into the sheep's femoral shaft by approaching the end of the bone from the knee joint and drilling an entry hole through the distal femoral growth plate. After we had finished the surgery, Dr. Biruk took the sheep to his home, where he and his children cared for them. At the end of their growth, x-rays and observation of the growth plates under the microscope showed little damage and minimal growth disruption. These studies were preliminary, so we did not yet recommend placement of the SIGN Pediatric Nail through the growth center of the femur at the knee.

We discussed our results with Dr. Raymond Liu, pediatric surgeon from Case Western Reserve University in Cleveland, OH. He had advised us during our initial sheep surgery in Ethiopia. He received a grant for a controlled study placing Schanz pins through the distal femoral growth center in a larger number of sheep. He and his resident orthopaedic surgeon, Dr. Derrick Knapik, presented their preliminary findings at the SIGN Conference in September 2016. They need to complete further studies of their samples before they can make conclusions about the consequences of placing an implant across the distal femoral growth plates of sheep, but preliminary results look promising.

Other preliminary findings from observing children's fractures treated with the SIGN Pediatric Fin Nails placed through the distal end of the femur by Mongolia surgeons include:

It is not necessary to design a new nail for a retrograde approach to pediatric femur fractures. The slot for the interlocking screw directs the screw above the physeal plate so that it can secure the fracture from rotating or sliding along the nail and still avoid damaging the growth plate.

The regular SIGN Fin Nail can be used if the canal is large enough. Apparently, in Mongolia, many canals are large enough, even in children as young as eight years old. The proximal slot is used for the interlocking screw in the fin nail. The fin nail's interlocking screw lies above the growth plate. With growth, the nail migrates toward the hip, which is away from the growth center, when the fracture has healed.

Fractures usually heal in three to five months. We are considering whether to suggest removing the nail, the interlocking screw, both, or neither. The nail and interlocking screw apparently do not affect the physeal plate, but we need further verification with long-term follow up.

The story of how SIGN's Implants have grown from a nail to treat tibia fractures to include implants designed for hip and pediatric femur fractures demonstrates our commitment to innovation and addressing the needs of our patient population. It is a challenge to temper the creative drive of our Mongolian colleagues to treat "unsolved" fractures with the sensitivity of Dr. Penaranda and his staff who consider the welfare of the individual patient first. The answer, I think, is to be contemplative and bold like the surgeons in Mongolia, Vietnam, Cambodia, Myanmar, and Afghanistan, but also document, combine, measure, and study our results through the SIGN Database so that we can learn from our mistakes and successes. This way we can continue to improve fracture care in the developing world—one patient at a time.

Chapter 8

SIGN Responds to Natural Disasters

Banda Aceh, Indonesia

The 2004 tsunami that leveled Banda Aceh on the island of Sumatra, Indonesia, killed at least 250,000 people. Many drowned as the wave rushed over them or pulled them out to sea when the waters receded. The survivors had soft-tissue injuries and fractures. Our Indonesian friends asked for help. We traveled to Jakarta, the capital city on the island of Java, to meet with them. Jeanne Dillner accompanied me on this trip, and I came to know her strong, forthright character. The Indonesian surgeons, concerned about her safety, wanted her to remain in Jakarta. They told us that a French volunteer had recently died in Banda Aceh. But Jeanne wasn't having any of it. She dismissed their anxiety with an immediate reply that reflected SIGN's resolve: "I came to help the injured in Banda Aceh."

As we traveled from the airport in Sumatra to the hospitals that were treating survivors, we noticed cars along the road that looked like they had been tossed into a giant blender. Actually, the vehicles had been rolled over and over, pulverized by the tsunami. Several miles from shore, in the middle of the city, a large ship stood upright—a memorial to the power of the tidal wave.

We met Dr. Azharuddin, who practiced orthopaedic surgery in Banda Aceh. We visited his clinic, where mud from the ocean surge

99

oozed from the books on his library shelf and covered the floor. After seeing his orthopaedic reference books covered in muck, I understood how Dr. Azharuddin could feel lost and alone. Nevertheless, we set to work doing SIGN Surgery together in mobile hospitals in Banda Aceh and later back in Jakarta.

A few years later, an earthquake occurred in central Java. This time orthopaedic residents from Jakarta accompanied us to the site. They visited the hospitals and prepared patients for SIGN Surgery. I assisted these residents and watched their skills performing the SIGN Technique improve quickly. A year later, another earthquake occurred. This time the surgeons from Indonesia treated the survivors with SIGN Implants without the need for outside help. Both the Indonesian surgeons and the SIGN Organization had grown in our abilities to respond to the challenges of a natural disaster.

This became apparent again in December 2016, when another earthquake occurred in Banda Aceh. One hundred people died and over 500 were injured. We contacted our friends in Indonesia, who asked only for SIGN Instruments and Implants, which we sent immediately. They were confident performing SIGN Surgery and did not request additional personnel.

Pakistan

SIGN expanded its capacities in Pakistan after a severe earthquake occurred in the mountains near Abbottabad in October 2005. Pakistani students from the United States and Pakistan organized the disaster response. They asked me to travel immediately to Islamabad with SIGN Equipment. When I came out of the airport in Islamabad, two men stood holding a card emblazoned with my name. They did not speak English and I did not speak Urdu, but we understood our common goal of treating earthquake survivors. We traveled together to Abbottabad, where I left the SIGN Equipment in a room supervised by a small number of Pakistani students. This was their command center. These young men were very cordial, spoke good English, and were extremely efficient. They organized rescue flights up into the mountains when they received distress calls. They had coordinated erection of a series of tents for triage in front of the hospital. We began surgical treatment in the hospital the next day.

I remember a Pakistani father whose son suffered a severe fracture of his proximal femur from the earthquake. He showed me his son's x-rays and followed me everywhere he could until we had scheduled his son for surgery. Caring for one's children is a universal trait. The surgery was successful.

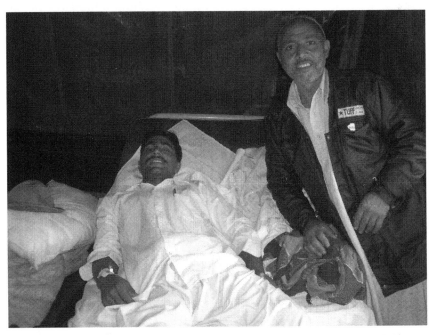

Father and son after successful SIGN Surgery for a fractured femur, which occurred in Pakistan earthquake.

One young orthopaedic surgeon in Abbottabad was very helpful in preparing the patients and assisting in surgery. He had earlier been dismissed from his orthopaedic residency in Islamabad and, at times, he expressed a hesitancy that reflected a loss of confidence. But I could see that he was very interested in learning orthopaedic surgery and was a hard worker. He showed great promise as a surgeon. One day the senior orthopaedic surgeon was late. The reticent young doctor and I stood scrubbed and waiting in the operating room. After a few minutes, standing over the anesthetized patient, I said, "Alam Zeb, this is our chance. Please proceed." I handed him the scalpel. He performed the surgery very well, placing the interlocking screws into the SIGN Implant on his first try. I could see his confidence rise. He just needed someone to hand him a knife and believe in him.

As the days after the earthquake wore on, we did many SIGN Surgeries but they became more difficult and took more time in the operating room. This was because the fractures were weeks old and began to heal in a shortened position. Muscle contractions due to the cold weather and prolonged pain pulled the fragments into malalignment. These fractures had to be brought out to length during the surgery or the patient would end up with a short leg and a permanent limp. The callous, or new bone, had to be removed, and the process of getting the bone out to length required more time than placing the nail and interlocking screws. If the surgery took twice as much time, we could only treat half as many patients each day. I realized we needed an instrument that would have a mechanical advantage stronger than a surgeon's hands to quickly pull the fracture apart and allow the nail to pass after the fragments were distracted. I decided that I would help our engineers design this instrument by returning home. Other distractors were already available, but they used pins that attached to bone fragments in order to pull the pieces apart. These pins had to be accurately drilled to avoid placement inside the canal, where they would block the path of the nail. Using these distractors was impractical because they require more incisions, longer operating time, and a C-arm for the surgeon to see pin placement and avoid obstructing the intramedullary canal.

On my way home from Pakistan to help the design team, I hired a car and driver to take me from Abbottabad to the airport in Islamabad. It was during Ramadan, the time of fasting, so we stopped to allow the driver to pray at the mosque and purchase fruit to eat when his fast ended that day. I had been invited by a Pakistani surgeon to stay overnight at the home of his relatives in Islamabad the night before the flight home. The surgeon had given me directions on a piece of paper, but neither my driver nor I could read them. Fortunately, our car stalled as we were searching for the house. As the car came to an unexpected halt, a man rushed out of his home to greet us. It turned out that we had broken down in front of the house that was our destination! When we parted, the driver and I gave each other the customary Pakistani hug. Both of us felt like destiny had brought us together in friendship just as it had delivered us to the correct address.

By the time I returned home, the SIGN Staff were completing the design of the distractor. Using their ingenuity and manufacturing abilities, the staff quickly produced the new product. Jeanne asked to accompany me, and three weeks later we returned to Pakistan with four SIGN Distractors. The distractors worked very well, and SIGN Staff continued to make improvements over the years. Innomed has now taken over the manufacturing and sells these distractors for a very reasonable price.

We made new friends during our second trip to Pakistan. Jeanne stayed in the home of a school principal, whose daughter was a medical student. I stayed in the home of an orthopaedic surgeon who entertained frequent visitors from around the world. I asked my host's daughter what she wanted to study in school. She said she wanted to be an astrophysicist. When I asked her why, she informed me that people always thought she was smart when she said she wanted to be an astrophysicist. I never knew what she really wanted to be, but she was smart. The hospitality shown to me in her home was humbling, gracious, and genuine. There are many good people throughout the world. I am grateful that my travels with SIGN have allowed me to know these good people. All people share a spark of humanity and the desire to make things better for those that cannot help themselves.

We traveled up the mountain roads to visit Muzaffarabad, the epicenter of the earthquake. The disaster struck at nine o'clock in the morning, when school was in session. Most of the buildings collapsed. Many schoolchildren died when the stone roofs fell on them. As we entered the rubble-filled town, we realized how dedicated the Pakistanis are to education. We saw groups of surviving children being instructed by their teachers on the side of the road.

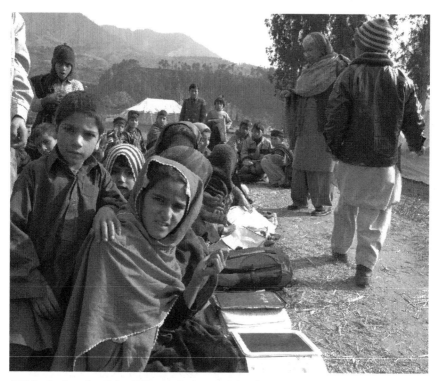

With their school buildings destroyed in the earthquake, these children used the road as a makeshift classroom.

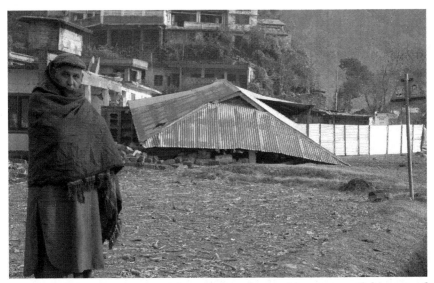

Earthquakes cause severe destruction, but with resourcefulness and perseverance, the Pakistani people have recovered and rebuilt their communities.

The SIGN Surgeons from Ghurki Trust Teaching Hospital in Lahore, Pakistan, were doing surgery in a modified shipping container near the epicenter of the earthquake. They were very well organized and had established an evacuation chain for spinal trauma and victims with more complex injuries. Over the years, I have seen many physicians operate in austere environments, as they did in Muzaffarabad, and I have come to respect the surgical skill and humanitarian outreach of SIGN Surgeons. Their collective experience and ability has grown to a point where they are frequently able to rely on each other rather than depend on intervention from the developed world. I can still hear Dr. Rizwan Akram from Ghurki Trust Teaching Hospital addressing surgeons from all over the developing world at our SIGN Conference in 2007. He was describing his experience treating Pakistani earthquake victims when he confidently offered to the audience, "If you have a disaster in your area, please call me. It is my duty to respond."

While we were still treating victims of the quake in Abbottabad, Professor A.A. Shah from Gilani Hospital Complex came to see us and invited us to visit his hospital. He had converted his private hospital to care for earthquake survivors. Some of the patients were in tents, but others had no shelter. During our SIGN Surgery together, I realized he was an excellent surgeon and I gave him a SIGN Set. He has used this SIGN Set to treat over 4,000 poor patients since the earthquake.

As SIGN's reputation grew in Pakistan, more hospitals requested our implants. The following letter from Dr. Mansoor Ilyas, the chief surgeon in a very busy hospital, demonstrates how SIGN had a positive effect in his country:

> *At the moment I am serving the Health Department of the Government of Balochistan as professor and head of the Orthopaedic Surgery Department at Bolan Medical College and the surgeon in chief at Sajid Hospital in Quetta. My whole career as a doctor is evolving around treating trauma.*
>
> *Back in 2009, while I was at Ghurki Hospital in Lahore for a symposium, I saw for the first time the SIGN Nailing cases, which were being done with manual reaming and without image intensifier. I was impressed, and especially I was much impressed by distal interlocking. That's when I decided to make contact with SIGN and was advised by Professor Zirkle to take a short training of the SIGN Nail with Professor Shahab in Peshawar, which I did in March 2009. On my return from Peshawar, we started the SIGN Nailing program in Sajid Hospital in Quetta under the kind guidance and support of Professor Zirkle.*
>
> *So far, I have done almost 300 cases, and none of them have had any complication. Not only the team*

under my supervision in Sajid Hospital but ultimately the masses of poor from Balochistan, Iran, and Afghanistan are the beneficiaries who are receiving high-quality hardware and a high standard of treatment, which are making their lives easier and more comfortable. All these endeavors are accomplishing the aim of SIGN to make the life of wounded people easier and more peaceful. On behalf of the SIGN Team and the poor people, we must extend our gratitude to Professor Lewis Zirkle.

There are now seven SIGN Programs in Pakistan. Dr. Ilyas and his Pakistani colleagues are doing excellent work. Many surgeons there have developed new treatments using SIGN Implants. I review their reports on the database, and I salute them for their results. It is an honor for me to work with the surgeons of Pakistan.

Haiti

SIGN came to Haiti after the terrible earthquake in January 2010. The quake caused many injuries because the epicenter was near Haiti's largest city and capital, Port-au-Prince. Dr. Scott Nelson, an orthopaedic surgeon who worked with SIGN in the Dominican Republic, was the first orthopaedic surgeon to fly to Port-au-Prince after the disaster. After he landed, the airport closed due to damages from the earthquake. Dr. Nelson led much of the initial medical response.

SIGN Headquarters in Washington teamed up with Medical Teams International of Portland, OR. They provided a small plane to fly Jeanne, me, and a shipment of SIGN Equipment from Florida to Haiti. We were joined by Dr. Ashok Shroff, an anesthesiologist from Kadlec Medical Center in Richland, WA. Dr. Ashok used his expertise in regional anesthesia to allow Haitian victims to undergo surgery without general anesthesia. The earthquake had destroyed most of the equipment necessary for general anesthesia, so Dr. Ashok's skills allowed us to operate on more earthquake victims. Jeanne worked as a nurse, sterilized the instruments, assisted in surgery, and did whatever was necessary to expedite patient care. We stayed in a house run by Dr. Joe and Linda Markee for Haiti Foundation of Hope. Both Joe, an OB/GYN doctor, and Linda trained at my alma mater, Duke University Medical Center. Haiti Foundation of Hope is an organization that provides medical care and schooling for Haitians.

All the men staying at Joe and Linda's house slept on the floor in one room. I didn't realize until that night how many men snored! One of our companions must have suffered from sleep apnea because he sounded like a large animal looking for a meal. I also didn't know, until then, that roosters crow through the night, as well as at sunrise. Planes landing at the nearby airport added to this cacophony and made sleep impossible, despite the hospitality of our hosts.

Different surgeons rotated through King's Hospital in Port-au-Prince. We worked there for four days. We used one headlamp to light the surgical site because electricity was not reliable. The surgeon who had the headlight became the chief surgeon, so we all scrambled to put it on first and be the primary surgeon for each case. The patients, traumatized by the earthquake, were afraid of aftershocks and did not want to sleep in any building. They lay, instead, on mattresses on the hill surrounding the hospital. When we made our preoperative rounds, I warned the patients that they would have to stay in the hospital after their surgeries until they were able to walk on crutches. Most patients, fearful to be under a roof that could collapse, hobbled outside to their mattresses after surgery on the same day.

We scheduled surgery for a 10-year-old boy with a severe fracture, but we had to cancel his case because a pregnant woman presented with a fractured femur and she was about to deliver her baby. When I told the boy that his case was postponed, he looked at me with a tear rolling down his cheek and said, "Don't forget about me!"

A doctor of obstetrics and gynecology from Massachusetts General Hospital in Boston, MA, was also volunteering at King's Hospital. So with one anesthetic, we combined the baby's delivery with surgery for the women's broken femur. After that, we fixed my teary friend's fracture. We didn't forget him.

Jeanne and I answered many calls requesting us to demonstrate SIGN Surgery and supply implants and instruments. We spent long hours visiting other Haitian hospitals and teaching SIGN Surgery. Dr. Scott Nelson, our colleague who came over from the Dominican Republic, called us from a community hospital treating Haitian earthquake victims. He had 12 patients with femur fractures that needed SIGN Implants. As an incentive for our help and our implants, he promised us nice warm beds after we completed the surgeries. We worked continuously for two days and two nights to fix the femur fractures. When we finished at four o'clock in the morning on the third day, Scott had disappeared. I finally found him in his "nice warm bed." He had fallen asleep on the concrete floor of the supply closet.

One of our pleasures in volunteering to assist disaster survivors is working with other physicians and orthopaedic surgeons. While working in Haiti, we met many dedicated physicians like Dr. Nelson. I was honored to work with the surgeons of the Shock Trauma Group from the University of Maryland Medical Center. They are one of the leading trauma hospitals in the United States. These surgeons and their staff provided excellent care to the earthquake victims in Haiti, and I learned a great deal from them.

After working with Dr. Nelson and catching some well-earned sleep, we received a distress call from the hospital ship USNS Comfort. The Navy ship was anchored outside Port-au-Prince in order to treat earthquake survivors on behalf of the US Government. The C-arm on the ship had broken, and they wanted to use the SIGN Instruments and Implants that did not require an image intensifier. The orthopaedic surgeon in charge was a friend of Dr. John Staeheli, my orthopaedic partner back home in Richland. The Navy made arrangements for us to fly by helicopter to the ship. After my Vietnam experience riding in helicopters, I was a little apprehensive about the flight to the ship. What a difference from Vietnam! The ride on the Navy helicopter was like cruising in an SUV; it was not the noisy, shaky ride of the Huey helicopters in Vietnam. We worked on the USNS Comfort for three nights. I was assigned to sleep in the enlisted men's bunk area. I have claustrophobia and the space was very crowded. It brought back the memories of sleeping at the Foundation of Hope house. I found an open area on the floor outside the room to sleep. I smiled as I nodded off, because this time I escaped the loud snores of a group of men. When we completed our work on the USNS Comfort, we left the SIGN Set on board. According to Ret. Captain Mike Bosse, the set is still there. It is ready to use to fix fractures if their C-arm breaks down again.

I flew from the ship back to mainland Haiti. I was walking up a hill lugging my duffel bag when a Navy commander asked if he could help. I was exhausted so I let him carry my gear. When he asked if he could do anything else for me, I answered in a tired voice, "You can get me out of here." The commander immediately arranged a flight for Jeanne and I on a C5 transport plane carrying Haitian people to Florida. We were strapped to the floor during takeoff and landing. After a week's rest, we were called back to Haiti to continue teaching SIGN Surgery and providing SIGN Instruments. Jeanne accompanied me on this and subsequent trips, and assisted in many surgeries. We make a great team.

The news media concentrated only on American surgeons who traveled to Haiti. The Haitian surgeons who spent long hours treating patients without complaining did not get proper credit. I asked them to write about their experiences during the earthquake. I then arranged for the American Academy of Orthopaedic Surgeons to publish the Haitian doctors' narratives in *AAOS Now*. The Haitian surgeons worked very hard and displayed great empathy for their fellow countrymen. Sadly, they had lost many of their nursing students when a dormitory collapsed during the earthquake.

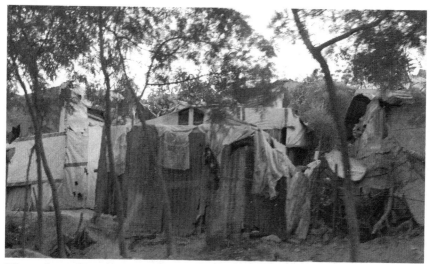

More than three years after the 2010 earthquake, many families still lived in structures cobbled together from rubble in Haiti.

Since the earthquake, SIGN has established 11 programs in Haiti. We have watched the surgical and diagnostic skills of these orthopaedic residents improve. The residency programs in Haiti now all use SIGN Implants and Instruments. Despite these accomplishments, Haiti is still struggling to recover from the devastation of the earthquake.

The government hospital infrastructure currently cannot handle the many road traffic accidents in Haiti. Frequent strikes of the personnel at these hospitals also delay patient care. Doctors Without Borders, often referred to by its French acronym MSF, remains very busy there. Mission hospitals also treat Haitian patients who are unable to receive care in the government institutions. The recent orthopaedic surgery graduates are excellent surgeons. Some of them are employed by MSF and mission hospitals. Unfortunately, their employment opportunities are limited in the government hospitals.

One group of recent orthopaedic graduates has organized to rotate to different hospitals and provide orthopaedic care when fractures arrive. We have provided them SIGN Instruments and Implants, and they have done many surgeries. Another group has rented an earthquake-proof clinic, which they would like to remodel to be a trauma hospital. They are looking for a loan to accomplish this. We have also provided this group with SIGN Equipment. These young doctors have plenty of patients, but there is no money to pay for their services. Many of them are forced to leave the country to seek fellowship training or lower level jobs just to feed their own families. Hopefully Haiti will find the resources to keep these surgeons home because seismologists predict that this poor island country will likely suffer more earthquakes and have more victims to treat.

Philippines

When Typhoon Haiyan struck the Philippines in 2014, local SIGN Surgeons organized an effective orthopaedic response. They established an evacuation chain, rotated medical personnel, and provided immediate medical care for typhoon survivors.

They already had many years of experience with SIGN Surgery and responding to natural disasters. All they needed was additional SIGN Implants, which we promptly sent.

Nepal

There were 11 SIGN Programs in Nepal when an earthquake struck in May 2015. The local surgeons mobilized the earthquake response and provided excellent care without outside help. Our headquarters responded to their requests for additional SIGN Sets and other orthopaedic equipment. Commercial implant companies also donated supplies, which we shipped to Nepal. Jeanne and I were working in Tanzania when the surgeons in Nepal asked us to visit a few weeks after the earthquake. We proceeded immediately to Nepal and were very pleased to see the quality of care that they provided. We visited four hospitals and operated in three of them while we were there. The Nepalese response to this disaster was excellent. At Nepal Orthopaedic Hospital we used a tent donated by the Canadian Army for our operating room. No post-operative infections occurred despite the challenges of keeping things sterile inside a tent. Afterward, the Nepalese surgeons organized a conference to discuss their reaction to the earthquake and identify ways to improve their response to a disaster in the future.

These more recent examples of local SIGN Surgeons handling natural disasters indicate to me that we can equalize fracture care in the world, even under the most challenging conditions. The best earthquake preparation is the SIGN Model of education plus donation of appropriate implants to surgeons in areas of potential disasters. These surgeons have shown themselves to be completely capable of handling disasters in their own country. Surgeons in the developing world are much like Alam Zeb, my young friend in Abbottabad; they just need someone to put the right instruments in their hands and believe in them.

Chapter 9

SIGN Encounters
Man-made Conflicts

The SIGN Nail was made to address the inequality of fracture care between industrialized countries and the developing world. The trends of more people moving to cities and more people traveling under motorized power has led to unprecedented suffering from road traffic accidents. As I previously described, natural disasters such as earthquakes and tsunamis have led to widespread suffering that is exacerbated by an inequality of care between the "haves" and the "have nots." Another factor constantly operating somewhere in the world that results in suffering and creates inequality—man-made conflict.

It is ironic that one of the first great paintings of the modern era, Francisco Goya's *The Third of May, 1808*, depicts the horror of war and demonstrates both the inequality and the suffering that results. My grandson, Harry, and I stood for a long time staring at this masterpiece hanging in the Prado Museum in Madrid, Spain. Goya depicts Napoleon's soldiers shooting Spanish peasants in order to avenge the death of French military killed during a local revolt. Harry and I focused on a kneeling peasant bathed in light from the soldiers' lantern and surrounded by fallen, bloodied, and terrified countrymen. Dressed in a simple white shirt, he raises his arms in a gesture of appeal or defiance. The firing squad are in darkness. Goya makes it obvious that they are about to shoot another target. To the executioners, the gesticulating peasant is no different from the bleeding pile of disposed victims in the foreground or those suffering as they wait in line in the background of the painting. To the soldiers, this special figure is not human. He is only something to dispose of.

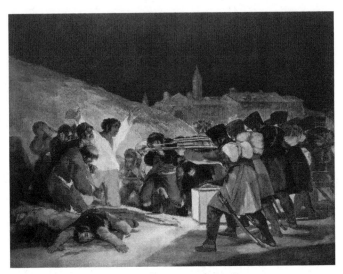

The Third of May 1808, by Francisco Goya

Violence and the reaction of brave people to violence is not confined to any one country or to any one group of people. Conflict increases inequality. The civilians caught between hostile forces are like the peasants in Goya's painting. They are human. They are each special and they endure the most violence, both emotionally and physically.

We have supplied SIGN Implants in many areas of conflict throughout the world. I have visited most of these areas and become very impressed with the surgeons who care for their people—both civilian and military.

This chapter is a tribute to the people who care for these civilians, often at great personal sacrifice.

Iraq

Dr. Rick Wilkerson, who served with the US Army in Iraq, asked me to travel to Iraq with him in 2007. We flew to northern Iraq from Amman, Jordan, and landed at night somewhere in the Iraqi desert. We rode a bus to Erbil, where we participated in a SIGN Conference attended by many surgeons from northern Iraq. We operated with Iraqi surgeons for six days, and I left two SIGN Sets with the surgeons so they could continue to treat the victims of war there.

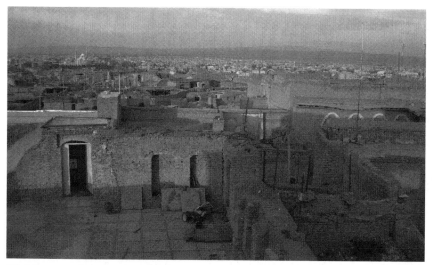

Eirbil, Iraq, is one of the oldest continually inhabited cities in the world.

Outside Erbil, a group of buildings sit on top of a dirt pile 100 feet high. We were told this was the oldest continually inhabited city in the world. I looked out over the countryside from a building on top of the dirt pile. Despite the war, the view of the sunset from the rooftop looked peaceful. As I admired the end of the day, I wondered why men continue to kill each other around this ancient city and around the world. I am puzzled by man's inhumanity to man. In Gaziantep, Turkey, I saw a similar structure, also reputed to be the oldest continually inhabited settlement in the world. Conflict is rampant in parts of the world that claim to have cradled civilization.

While I was in Iraq, we drove around in a small Suzuki. A military convoy passed us. I wondered who was safer: the soldiers in their armored vehicles or us in our little Suzuki. I had the same feeling when Jeanne and I were walking between hospitals in Afghanistan in 2007 and 2008. The choice is to blend in or stand out with guns and armor.

Dr. Gordon Hsieh, my partner at Northwest Orthopaedic Associates in Richland, WA, had been stationed in Iraq with Col. Jim Ficke. When Col. Ficke contacted Gordon and requested a SIGN Set to treat civilian casualties in Mosul, Iraq, we tried to accommodate him. To stay under the postal weight limits, we sent a few instruments and implants at a time through the Army/Air Post Office. After the US forces withdrew from Mosul, we continued the SIGN Program in a civilian hospital until the city was taken over by ISIS. At the time I am writing this chapter, US-led forces are once again fighting to retake Mosul. We are looking for ways to help the wounded civilians there.

Surgeons from Sulaymaniyah, in the Kurdish area of Iraq, attended the SIGN Conference at our headquarters in 2016. They asked if we would start a SIGN Program in their hospital. They also presented me with a research proposal by Professor Barawi at the University of Sulaymaniyah. Orthopaedic surgeons bond together with their common interest in surgery even when they come from very different backgrounds. This diversity is one of the strengths of the SIGN Family.

Major Matthew Martin, MD, a trauma surgeon from Portland, OR, and colleague of Dr. Rich Gellman, was stationed in Iraq. Dr. Gellman knew that we wanted to provide SIGN to treat the civilians and others injured in the battle for Mosul. The International Committee of the Red Cross has a hospital there, but they were not stabilizing fractures, so patients had no place to get definitive care. Dr. Martin was stationed with Dr. Doug Adams, an orthopaedic surgeon. We communicated and made arrangements to ship a SIGN Set to their unit in Baghdad. That are performing SIGN Surgery now with great skill for the civilians injured in Mosul.

Afghanistan

Dr. David Templeman, a volunteer trauma surgeon, Jeanne, and I first traveled to Afghanistan in 2007 at the request of Jerry Daly, who was the administrator of Wazir Akbar Khan Hospital, the largest civilian hospital in Kabul. Sixteen percent of their injured patients traveled part of the journey to the hospital by donkey. Can you imagine the pain elicited at the fracture site with each donkey jolt? Movement of a fracture is very painful.

The orthopaedic residents and staff in Wazir Khan Hospital were very interested in learning better ways to treat their patients with fractures. They asked many questions as we discussed the different types of surgical treatment of fractures. This was similar to conversations in which I have participated throughout the world. We discussed the difference between plating of the femur and using the IM nail interlocking screw fixation, which is more difficult but leads to better results. Our conversation motivated the residents to research and write a paper showing the superiority of fracture treatment using the SIGN Nail compared with using plates. Orthopaedic surgery residents throughout the world are very similar—they all have a thirst for learning in order to provide the best care for their patients.

Patients in Wazir Khan Hospital who had difficult orthopaedic problems and those who did not accept the surgeon's recommendations were placed on a remote ward. The nurses took us to the remote ward in order to meet a man who fell in a well. The wells in Afghanistan are not enclosed. The man had fallen in the well at night. He had severe fractures of his heels, and the surgeons advised him to have amputation. He refused and was placed in this remote ward, along with other patients who had little hope of recovery from their fractures. Prostheses for amputees were not available in most of Afghanistan. I examined him, reviewed his x-rays, and felt that I could help him save his damaged heels. I asked the chief of orthopaedics to operate on this patient with me, but the chief didn't say yes or no. He continued to schedule different cases for us. He wanted me to teach his surgeons orthopaedic procedures, such as the reconstruction of the anterior cruciate ligaments in the knee. I finally told him that this man must be operated as the first case, and then we would do knee reconstruction surgery. I'm happy to say that both salvaging the little man's feet and the knee reconstruction surgery were successful.

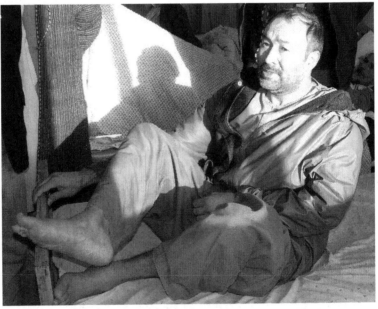

This man fell into a well in Afghanistan, resulting in severe fractures to both feet. These fractures were reduced and fixed.

Every day, on our way to the hospital, we would pass approximately 10 men squatting on top of a wall. I assumed they were relatives of hospital patients. During my travels, I have learned that people in different cultures express themselves with their eyes in a variety of ways. In some cultures, it is impolite to look a stranger in the eye, but in Afghanistan we were often met with piercing stares, especially by these 10 men. After we operated on the little man's heels, the squatters softened their facial expressions. On one occasion, I saw slight smiles on their lips. Our gesture to provide quality care to relieve the suffering of the poor man who tumbled into a well bridged a gap of culture, religion, and prejudice. Scowls turned into smiles because we recognized the common spark of humanity in all of us.

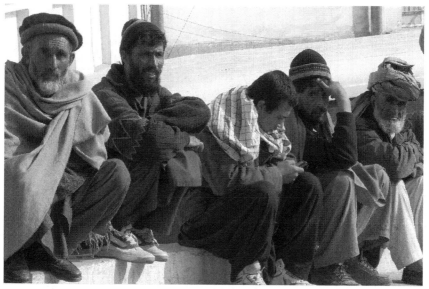

Men sitting outside Wazir Khan Hospital in Afghanistan.

The National Military Hospital was two blocks away from Wazir Khan Hospital, in Kabul. In 2007 this busy hospital treated both civilians and military and was the largest military hospital in Afghanistan. The military surgeons all wanted to participate in SIGN Surgery, and they proved to be very skilled. Dr. Ismail Wardak is the SIGN Representative in Afghanistan. He advises us about which hospitals can receive and use the SIGN Implants and

SIGN Techniques. The chosen surgeons learn SIGN Technique from Dr. Wardak and his staff.

Many Afghanistan surgeons have trained in Russia, where, in the 1950s, Gavriil Abramovich Ilizarov pioneered a unique method of correcting bone deformity and treating fractures that had not healed. Ilizarov used circular frames and wires based on the stability of a spoked bicycle wheel. His techniques are still used today.

Dr. Wardak has applied the principles of the Ilizarov technique to design and popularize a treatment of both kneecap and arm fractures. Other Afghan surgeons have also developed modifications of the external fixation technique of Ilizarov. Surgeons throughout Afghanistan use Dr. Wardak's innovation. They presented their positive results with this technique at the second and third International SIGN Conference in Kabul in 2015.

One of our patients at the Afghan Army National Hospital had fractures of both tibias that had not healed for years, despite several operations. The patient's son was a doctor in this hospital, so Dr. Wardak wanted to use the best implant available for the surgery. He asked that we use SIGN Implants and Technique to stabilize the tibia fractures. I assisted Dr. Wardak in performing SIGN Surgery for both tibias. Halfway through the first procedure, the patient looked up at Jeanne, who was at the head of the operating room table, and said, "I love the United States." During our second trip to Afghanistan, a year later, Dr. Wardak said that someone wanted to see us. We went into a hallway and saw our former patient walking down the stairs without a limp. He had lost weight and looked very healthy. Results like this elicit the ecstasy of doing SIGN Surgery. I also get a similar pleasure watching surgeons in developing countries accomplish difficult surgery using the SIGN System with minimal equipment.

Return to Afghanistan

In 2008 we were asked by the military surgeons to return to Afghanistan. We operated for a week with them and then took part in a SIGN Conference. The conference room was filled with orthopaedic surgeons from all parts of Afghanistan. I was humbled to learn that these surgeons had come over treacherous roads to attend this conference. The surgeons were very enthusiastic and formed the Afghanistan Orthopaedic Association and established the Journal of Afghanistan Orthopaedics.

One of the anesthesiologists who worked with us at the military hospital was also an Afghan military general. The general and I developed a mutual respect for each other, perhaps because we had similar limps due to our arthritic knees. I knew his attitude warmed toward me when he observed that I was an active assistant, helping the Afghan surgeons do difficult surgery, rather than doing the surgery myself. After the last surgery as we were leaving, I wanted to say goodbye to the Afghan general, but he could not be found. Reluctantly, I started walking from the hospital. The weather was cold, and the snow fell in tiny ice balls. I had walked about 200 yards when I heard someone shout that the general was coming. I turned back to the hospital and saw him shuffling my way. As we both limped toward each other, I thought of the Hollywood western, *High Noon*, in which two young men approach each other in the blazing heat of mid-day ready to draw their pistols in a duel. I chuckled at the contrast in the weather, the gaits, and the reasons for approach between the actors in the movie and us two old men wishing each other farewell.

Since bidding the general goodbye, SIGN has received and granted many requests for implants from military and civilian hospitals throughout Afghanistan. Dr. Wardak has trained the majority of the surgeons who are using SIGN Implants there.

Dr. Wardak has continued to advise us about which hospitals in Afghanistan should receive SIGN Instruments and Implants. Here is a letter from Dr. Wardak:

As a SIGN Surgeon, my team and I treated almost 1,000 cases in two centers in the past four years. I also tried my best to spread SIGN Programs all over Afghanistan, and now we have more than 15 programs. In the last four years, after having observed minimal complications, easy procedure, and trustable fixation, I decided to treat one of our family members using SIGN.

My brother's wife, 40 years old, complained of pain in her right hip for a month. When we got an x-ray, she had a deformed hip joint due to a fracture 30 years ago. The affected limb was three centimeters short because the angle of the femoral neck to the shaft had changed.

Subtrochanteric wedge osteotomy (cutting the bone, so it will heal in a position to change the forces and length on the leg) was the best solution for realignment and restoration of normal length. For fixation of such osteotomy site, there are so many ways and different implants to use, such as DHS, plates, nails, and even external fixation, but we selected the SIGN Interlocking System.

Some say not to operate on your close relative, but for me, as a surgeon, I pretend all my patients are my close relatives, and during surgery, there is no difference for me. I used a SIGN Nail for the first time for such case in Afghanistan, and I think it's new for other types of operations. As the fixation was so strong, there was no need for a supplementary cast or brace, so we allowed her to walk with crutches.

Now she's doing well, and our family is happy. On behalf of my family, I'm thankful for SIGN.

Dr. Michelle Foltz has visited Afghanistan many times and suggested we provide SIGN Implants to the hospital in Mazar-e-Sharif. She has also worked in two hospitals run by the Italian charity, EMERGENCY. She has worked in both EMERGENCY hospitals, one in Kabul and the other in Helmand Province, where we provide SIGN Implants. Dr. Foltz is a tough woman. She has shown as much bravery as any male orthopaedic surgeon in her travels around the world.

Third Visit to Afghanistan

Our third trip to Afghanistan in November 2015 was prompted by an invitation from Dr. Wardak to participate in the third Afghan SIGN Conference. He was concerned because the Afghanistan medical establishment was not receiving help from US military, except for transportation of patients. Many non-governmental organizations that provided medical assistance had also left Afghanistan when US combat troops were drawn down beginning in 2012.

When we arrived, we were given sleeping accommodations in the Central Afghan National Army Hospital. At five o'clock in the morning, helicopters began arriving carrying injured patients. The helicopter sounds flooded me with memories of treating war casualties during my US Army days in Vietnam. I realized that these helicopters were likely transporting soldiers wounded in battle. The hospital had stopped treating civilians, despite increasing numbers of road traffic accidents, so that it could concentrate its limited resources on military casualties.

Two hundred people filled the conference room for the third Afghan SIGN Conference. I was once again impressed by the bravery of the Afghanistan surgeons who had traveled many miles over insecure roads to attend the conference. The orthopaedic surgeons from Kunduz had encountered shooting from the Taliban on their journey. These resourceful surgeons had left their car, walked around the fighting, and hitched a ride the rest of the way to Kabul in order to make it to the conference.

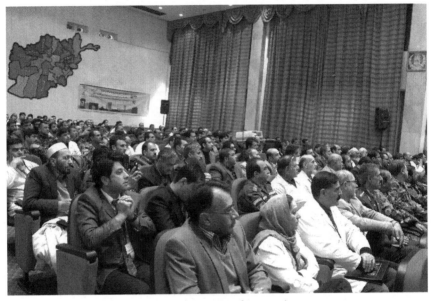

Surgeons at the third Afghan SIGN Conference in 2015.

Since this conference, we have started new SIGN Programs in Kunduz and Khost. We talked with an MSF surgeon who worked in a hospital that was inadvertently destroyed by helicopter bombs. He will work with the surgeons in Kunduz in our new SIGN Program. Drs. Wardak and Siawash taught the SIGN Technique to the surgeons in Kunduz and Kabul.

The Afghan conference presentations described the treatment of different traumatic injuries using the SIGN System, as well as other topics of general interest. Several series of patients with patella and olecranon fractures who were treated with Dr. Wardak's device again showed excellent results.

The Afghan surgeons were wonderful hosts. Twice we traveled to surgeons' homes for meals with their families. The men and women ate separately, as is the custom. The children were eager to tell us their hopes and dreams for the future. Many talked about the occupations they hoped to enter, and they showed great determination to achieve their goals despite the limitations imposed by the war. I realized that the Afghanistan surgeons and families share similar hopes about the future as American surgeons and families.

During our stay, the Afghan military provided a commando as our personal bodyguard. He carried an assault rifle with him and was very attentive to our security. One morning we were taken to President Ghani's office where Dr. Wardak, Jeanne, and I were presented the Allama Sayed Jamaluddin Afghan Medal, Afghanistan's second-highest civilian honor. We accepted the honor on behalf of the entire SIGN Family. We found President Ghani to be very engaging, and we had a pleasant interchange before and after the ceremony. He had been a student in the American Field Service Intercultural Programs and studied in Oregon. Jeanne grew up in Oregon, so she had some common background with him. President Ghani is an anthropologist; he is very honest and is doing his best for the people of Afghanistan. I admire him for returning to Afghanistan to help his people. This trip enhanced our commitment to Afghanistan. The surgeons face insecurity every day but are trying to live a normal life with their families and take good care of their patients. They want more education and more SIGN Implants. They want to provide treatment of pelvic fractures, and we have provided them with education, instruments, and implants.

South Sudan

Conflict has been increasing in South Sudan since the country separated from Sudan in 2011. Conflict brings chaos, and chaos has led to corruption. The government has received grant money for maternal and child health care, but none for surgical care.

Dr. Akau Aguto and Dr. James Alfonse work in the capital city at Juba Teaching Hospital and provide most of the orthopaedic care in the country. We have visited Juba twice and have been impressed with their dedication as well as the difficult conditions in South Sudan. These men do excellent surgery.

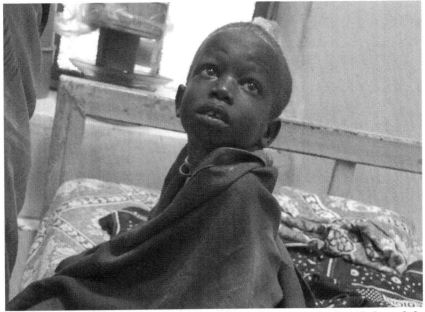

Children, like this girl from South Sudan, do not understand the adult conflict surrounding them, though they are often casualties.

The last time we were there, two young interns, Dr. Mapuor Mading and Dr. Festo Lado, were extremely busy taking care of many patients on the surgical wards. They were very eager to learn and wanted more orthopaedic training so they could help their people. The patient load is overwhelming, and government support—or lack of support—is frustrating, but these interns were determined to help their people, just as their colleagues were in Afghanistan. They requested help from SIGN. We gave them books, but they wanted more. They wanted to enroll in an orthopaedic residency program to *really* learn more orthopaedic surgery. Since both spoke English well, we sought formal orthopaedic residencies for them. Dr. Mapuor is now an orthopaedic resident at the Muhimbili Orthopaedic Institute in Dar es Salaam, Tanzania. His expenses and tuition are paid for by Elaine and Nate Ballou of West Richland, WA. Dr. Festo is currently an orthopaedic resident at Tenwek Hospital, in Kenya. After their orthopaedic surgery training, they both plan to return to work in South Sudan.

During a conference at Muhimbili Orthopaedic Institute, Tanzania, I saw Dr. Mapuor enthusiastically demonstrating the SIGN Technique to other surgeons from East Africa. He based his explanation on his experience doing SIGN Surgery at Juba Teaching Hospital. Dr. Mapuor is as tall as he is bright. He is a member of the Dinka tribe, who have the longest tibias in the world. Tibia, femur, and humerus lengths are very important to supplying the proper size SIGN Implants to different programs. We have empiric knowledge of bone hardness and length of patients throughout the world, due to the SIGN Database and personal experience.

During our first trip to South Sudan, we were accompanied by Randy Huebner and Joel Gillard, both engineers who have played an integral role in the development of instruments and implants for SIGN. They organized the surgical supply room and repaired operating room equipment in Juba using their Leatherman multi-tools. They left these useful tools with the operating room staff when they returned home. On our second visit to South Sudan, Dr. Michael Mara, chief of orthopaedics at Kijabe Hospital in Kenya, accompanied us. He noted a deficiency in anesthesia at Juba and was determined to organize a program to teach anesthetists from South Sudan in his hospital back in Kenya.

South Sudan is full of tragedies. We saw a large boat hit a rock and tip over into the Nile River. The boat was filled with refugees and all of their belongings. Fortunately, another boat came to rescue the passengers, but most of their belongings were lost. We saw many refugees in camps along the banks of the Nile, another result of man's inhumanity to man.

We received the following letter from Dr. Mapuor in mid-2016:

Juba is one of the oldest centers of the government since its establishment in 1922 as a small town by Greek traders. On July 9, 2011, it became the national capital city of the newly independent country of South Sudan. Juba Teaching Hospital (JTH), which was a military barracks in early 1923, is now the only center for services in the whole country. As I have been working in JTH since April 2011, I learnt from my seniors that with SIGN, we could save lives.

The hospital received approximately 450 to 500 and admitted 60 to 80 patients a day from both within Juba and from all around the country. People walked for days to Juba, and relatives carried their sick patients on their shoulders to Juba hospital. For example, on your visit in May 2013, you operated on a blind man with fracture femur who had been carried for two days by his relatives to JTH to get his fracture fixed.

Dr. Akau has worked hard to teach me the basic orthopaedic principles of fracture management such that I can go down to the far towns from Juba where there are patients who can't make it to Juba.

In May 2012, a few months after separation from the North, war erupted at the border between the government of South Sudan and the Khartoum (Sudan) government, and the government had to send me, my friend Festo, and one general surgeon to the town of Benito to treat the wounded civilians and soldiers. Then, after that, I was able to visit many state hospitals to treat trauma cases and advise patients with complicated cases to be sent to Juba to Dr. Akau.

On Dec. 15, 2013, when war broke out in Juba City and spread down to the towns of South Sudan, JTH overflowed with wounded patients. No medical personnel had a rest for almost three days. After that, I had to travel to the state hospitals where wounded patients were. I traveled to Rumbek State Hospital in April 2014 where 71 wounded patients were. I worked there for 21 days. In May, the African Medical and Research Foundation took me to Wau Teaching Hospital and Kuajok State Hospital. To these hospitals I carried with me external fixators which the SIGN Program had provided to JTH.

My mission to those hospitals was not only to treat patients, but to teach the nurses and medical doctors who had no chance to be in JTH to get the training I got from Dr. Akau, Dr. James, and the SIGN visitors.

Dr. Akau, the chief surgeon at Juba Teaching Hospital, spent 16 years in Norway and returned to South Sudan six years ago to help his people. His family is still in Norway. The other surgeon, Dr. James Alfonse, is a general in the South Sudan Army.

I want to honor Drs. Mapuor, Festo, Akau, and James as examples of real heroes—the surgeons who remain and work in their countries to help their people. Dr. Mapuor informed me that he is not yet a hero, but he is training to be one.

Conditions in Juba Teaching Hospital are becoming more urgent. The government now does not supply oil to power the electricity for the hospital on a consistent basis. Dr. Akau said that they do not get enough power during the day to run the sterilizer. He noted that the anesthesia machines and the lights in the operating room have stopped working at crucial times. Joel Gillard contacted Leatherman Tool Group, who donated LED Lenser headlamps that surgeons could use for lighting during surgery. I purchased spinal needles and spinal anesthetic that could be used so general anesthesia was not necessary. We had operated this way in Haiti. The SIGN System does not require any power, so Juba Teaching Hospital surgeons can continue to treat their patients.

Dr. Mapuor plans to return to practice in his hometown Rumbek, South Sudan. The hospital there does not have orthopaedic equipment, so SIGN is working to provide this equipment in addition to the SIGN Equipment. Dr. Mapuor will finish his residency in Dar es Salaam in September 2017 and will spend three months with another SIGN Surgeon, Dr. Sami Hailu, learning pelvic fracture surgery in Ethiopia before returning home.

Syria

I was invited by Dr. Sam Attar, a member of the Syrian American Medical Society from Baltimore, MD, to teach a SIGN Conference for Syrian surgeons in Gaziantep, Turkey in 2013. Dr. Sam had operated in Aleppo on two occasions. As in Afghanistan, surgeons in conflict areas must take risks to attend conferences to increase their orthopaedic surgery skills. The surgeons from Syria evoked feelings of humility, anger, and sympathy in me as they told their stories. They convinced me that SIGN Implants were needed in Syria. Their hospitals were located in the basements of buildings, because barrel bombs were frequently dropped on hospitals. The Syrian physicians who worked in these hospitals were labeled terrorists by the Syrian government, as were their families. While many surgeons had sent their families to refugee camps in neighboring countries, they had chosen to remain in Syria to treat the numerous injuries resulting from the conflict. Most of the injuries they treated resulted from sniper shots, bombs, and missile attacks, and many women and children were injured.

As I listened to their stories, I watched their faces reflect despair and helplessness as well as determination to continue their patient care in Syria. One doctor from Damascus told of being overcome by chlorine gas poisoning that had infested the clothes of his patients. He passed out and was given atropine to revive him, but he was blind for seven days. Although he continues to be fatigued, he had walked 40 kilometers to the conference to learn more about treating victims of gas poisoning and SIGN Surgery. Sadly, one of his walking partners had stepped on a mine and was killed. This brave physician had to walk back along this same route. Before he started back, he described his fellow surgeons as ducks on the water—calm on top, but paddling furiously below the surface.

Emmanuel Kant writes that every man has absolute value. Absolute value of a human being does not depend on nationality, family, gender, distance from us, or any other distinction. The value of every person is not relative but absolute. This is reflected in the vision statement of SIGN: Creating equality of fracture care throughout the world. Every person must be valued and cared for, no matter where they are. Even though these Syrian surgeons are too psychologically traumatized to offer solutions to the conflict, they seek assistance to help them treat their patients. We must respond, and we will always respond to future requests from distressed people.

At the Gaziantep conference, we discussed fracture treatment using SIGN Technique and distributed two sets of SIGN Implants and Instruments to the Syrian American Medical Society, as well as other implants from five suitcases I had brought. I felt very inadequate because we did not have enough SIGN Sets for all the hospitals that needed them. I committed to sending at least three more SIGN Sets, which we have now done.

Surgeons form bonds because of their common orthopaedic interest and desire to provide the best care for their patients. I felt guilty leaving these surgeons as they struggled emotionally and physically to treat the many injuries of their compatriots caused by ruthless, needless conflict. We Americans have the luxury to go about our daily activities without risk of random gunshot wounds and bombs dropped indiscriminately on hospitals and schools. That's why we must pay it forward and provide as much assistance as possible to our fellow human beings in need.

We live in a time of great inequity at home and abroad, as Samantha Power, former US Ambassador to the United Nations, says in her book, *A Problem from Hell: America and the Age of Genocide*. Power tells the story from many aspects: the people who suffer, the people who create the suffering, and the reaction of other countries, especially the United States.

The history of Syria, Afghanistan, Iraq, and South Sudan is fraught with conflict. We must not just read about it—we must act to alleviate the suffering. The cost of war is borne by the innocent, many of whom have no stake in the conflict. Current wars precipitate post-traumatic stress syndrome in those who have been in combat.

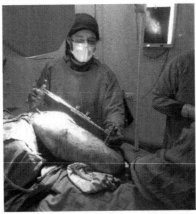

*Surgeons in Aleppo, Syria, are performing SIGN
Surgery in the midst of conflict and bombing.*

Here is a letter we received from a surgeon practicing in Syria:

Dear Dr. Zirkle,

We thank your great efforts in helping our people. We always need your advice and comments in order to improve the quality of our work.

Nowadays in Aleppo are very catastrophic as all the bombs of the world are falling on people, buildings, trees, animals... We don't know how to stop this crazy bloodstream of nonstop massacres every day, as if the people here don't deserve to live in peace.

Again, thanks for your help.

Why include conflict areas in the story of SIGN? The story of SIGN is about reducing suffering in the developing world by providing fracture care that is as effective as the care in developed countries.

Man-made conflicts have the power to create the kind of suffering depicted in Goya's masterpiece. Visits to Iraq, Afghanistan, South Sudan, and Gaziantep, Turkey, have taught us how extensively innocent civilians are victimized by the conflicts there and how bravely their physicians sacrifice to help them. In the hands of local surgeons, SIGN Implants can be a tool for reducing the tragic consequences of this violence. It is our duty to assist these surgeons who remain in their countries to treat the wounded.

SIGN is well-suited to support surgeons in conflict areas because the SIGN Instruments are designed to stabilize fractures in austere environments, and we provide the implants at no cost to the patients in need. My heroes are those who care for the injured in conflict. They quietly make this decision to help those whom Goya painted, those who are on their knees facing and suffering from the dark weapons of war.

Chapter 10

Creativity

"The real voice of discovery consists not in seeking new landscapes but in looking with new eyes" —Marcel Proust

"Looking with new eyes" was the theme of the 2016 Annual SIGN Conference. The SIGN Family is composed of surgeons of many diverse cultures. We have bonded due to our common interest in providing the best care possible to poor patients, and our diverse experiences enable us to see past our own biases and find new solutions. Many of the clinical studies presented by the surgeons shared new ideas for treating patients using SIGN Equipment. Most of their presentations ended with a question stimulated by their study.

These questions were prompted by the previous year's conference, where we talked about the book *A More Beautiful Question*, by journalist and innovator Warren Berger. He discusses the power of inquiry to spark breakthrough ideas, which is linked with Proust's "looking with new eyes." The synergy of looking with new eyes and asking questions is essential for SIGN Surgeons. We must substitute innovation for the instruments which United States surgeons are accustomed to being available for every surgery.

Creativity has played an important role in the journey of SIGN. This creativity manifests itself throughout the SIGN Family of surgeons, nurses, engineers, and staff.

The creative surgeons must first understand the connection between mechanical principles of fracture stabilization and biological factors related to fracture healing. The creativity of the SIGN Family and reports submitted to the SIGN Surgical Database provide validation for the SIGN System and Surgeons. There are many reports in the database, which we review to make algorithms for treating particular fractures. Surgeons can use these algorithms to decide which approach for each surgery, type and length of nail, and other decisions. Each surgeon must consider his ability, equipment available, and many other aspects to provide the best care for his patients. Many SIGN Surgeons follow the game plan as listed below.

- **Question conventional wisdom.** Decision makers in orthopaedic surgery often make statements and soon everyone repeats them. These are the experts in conventional wisdom. While I respect their wisdom, we question this especially because our surgeons work in austere conditions not faced by these decision makers.

- **Celebrate diversity.** Scott Page, in his book *The Difference: How the Power of Diversity Creates Better Groups, Firms, Schools, and Societies*, mathematically shows that diversity trumps ability. We celebrate not only the diversity between SIGN Surgeons but the diversity between people of different talents and ideas. When I have an idea, I "throw out the net." I send this idea to many people and they respond according to their bias and experience.

- **Contemplate frequently.** Take 10-minute breaks to exercise or walk and think. This is good for general health and the contemplation allows us to gather, evaluate, and synthesize new information. Contemplation allows us to be alert to sentinel events that may change our ideas. Contemplation can be directed backward, as just described, or forward because we should have no restraints. Contemplation should involve divergent thinking based on undirected thought and convergent thinking where we analyze and refine our thoughts. Changing locations such as traveling to SIGN Programs is a stimulus for contemplation.

The process of technological development involves collaboration between peers and those who go before us. We can see this in the evolution of intramedullary fixation. Every generation of surgeons takes credit for their contributions and, if we are not careful, we can trick ourselves into believing we did the most important part—like the rooster who believes that his crowing brings the sun up. The reality is that each contribution has to follow previous work. We do stand on the shoulders of giants from whom we learned a great deal. We're learning a great deal from the SIGN Surgical Database, but we must consider that many people have contributed to the database, and creative diversity is very important.

When creativity starts flowing, it is like a sailboat in a high wind. The moment when the hull lifts out of the water and there is no drag is the creative "aha." We then enjoy the ride but continue to steer the boat.

Chapter 11

Voices of SIGN

Physicians have a responsibility and an obligation to use their training and talents to treat patients in need. In his novel, *The Stranger*, French Nobel laureate Albert Camus suggests that we must speak for those who cannot speak for themselves, unlike his narrator Meursault, who has no empathy. In *The Plague*, Camus tells the story of Doctor Rieux and journalists who value moral responsibility over happiness when they remain in the city to treat victims of bubonic plague. I see the same moral virtues in surgeons in areas of conflict who stay in their country to take care of their people. They put their lives in danger every day. These surgeons are my heroes.

SIGN Surgeons consider that it is their obligation to provide equality of fracture care to patients with high energy injuries in developing countries. The photo of "The Man in the Bed" that hangs on the wall at SIGN Headquarters next to a quotation from Abraham Heschel from his book, *Who is Man?*: "Over and above personal problems, there is an objective challenge to overcome inequality, injustice, helplessness, and suffering. To accept the challenge, I must answer these questions: What is expected of me? What is demanded of me?"

This chapter contains the voices of SIGN. These voices are the words of surgeons who describe the joy they find in treating patients. I have not named surgeons in conflict areas due to security reasons.

Turbulent Emotions

In January 2017 we received the following email from a surgeon in Afghanistan. It is an example of the turbulent emotions SIGN Surgeons endure in areas of conflict when they must consider their obligations to their families and their patients. In 2015, we started a new SIGN Program in Kunduz after the MSF Hospital had been mistakenly bombed. In the chapter about man-made conflict, I discussed his story of determination to come to the SIGN Conference in Kabul to request a SIGN Set.

Dear friends,

I'm sorry I have not been able to keep in touch with you and reply sooner. I have been unwell for the past few weeks and have been in Kabul attending to some important personal matters. In my absence, I have given the responsibility of all SIGN Operations to my colleagues, orthopaedic specialists. I will be returning to Kunduz soon and will tend to any issues or problems personally.

Kunduz is in an extremely bad state. Currently, it is in a state of war, and almost on a nightly basis, there are attacks on the city. There is fighting during the day, and it only gets worst at night. The son of a fellow doctor, who is a close friend, was kidnapped a couple of weeks ago, and the boy is still missing. I am a family man and have children myself and have come to Kabul to settle them down here. I plan on returning to Kunduz, because nothing brings me more satisfaction and joy than doing what we do, no matter what the situation. After reviewing and catching up with the situation there, I will be able to get back to you in a useful manner.

The 10% Fund

In the following email of December 8, 2016, from Nigeria, Dr. Anire Bafor tells us about a fund he established to help his indigent patients pay for treatment.

I trust that everything is going well. I believe I've been able to gather the information I was looking for through networking. So far, I've been able to determine that there are 16 SIGN Programs in Nigeria, 15 active and one inactive. All program managers are on WhatsApp [a messaging application for smartphones] group I created called the Nigerian SIGN Forum.

The intention of this group is to foster collaboration amongst ourselves, network for educational and research purposes, and keep the SIGN Philosophy alive in Nigeria. The idea has been very receptive here.

I am attaching two pictures to this mail. One is a picture of me and the very first beneficiary from my '10% fund.' I still haven't decided on a name for the foundation, but I won't let waiting for an appropriate name delay my helping hand. The patient is sitting on the bed, and his father is standing next to him. He had fractures of his right femur and both tibiae, as well as his left radius and ulna. They are very indigent. He had SIGN Nailing for his right femur, and both tibiae, as well as plate and screw fixation of his forearm fractures with plates and screws donated by me. From the fund I was able to pay for his surgery fees and all other hospital charges. The alternative, which they were going to take, was to go to the native bonesetters. I'm just glad I was able to make a difference in his life with the great help of SIGN.

The father wrote a beautiful letter of thanks. I will scan and send this at a later date.

It is my incontrovertible belief that acts of kindness make the world a much better place.

The 10% fund is an idea I came up with after many years of being painfully frustrated by seeing patients who want orthodox treatment but can't afford it. I decided to do something about it. For a few months now, I have been putting aside 10% of my earnings from all sources. It is from this source that I'm able to take care of medical bills of indigent patients. Hopefully, it'll grow to be a much bigger project so that more people can benefit.

Once again I want to express my gratitude to Dr. Zirkle and all of the wonderful people working at SIGN for the divine work you guys are doing. You guys are a constant source of inspiration to us. God bless you all immensely.

Queen of the SIGN Nail

In the following story, surgeons at Al-Khidmat Al-Hajeri Hospital in Quetta, Pakistan, tell us about a little girl who gained not only surgeries, but new names.

When Fatimah visited us the first time, she was eight years old and suffering from osteogenesis imperfecta, commonly known as brittle bone disease. The disease caused her right femur to fracture. Fatimah was treated with the standard SIGN IM Nail which enabled her leg to heal.

In Urdu, the language spoken by Fatimah's Pakistani family, Eman means faith. After her recovery, her parents changed her name to Eman Fatimah.

144

Eman's struggles with brittle bone disease are not over. At age 11, she recently broke her left humerus. The surgeons at Al-Khidmat Al-Hajeri Hospital treated this fracture with a SIGN Fin Nail.

Abirah means strong and powerful in Urdu, and her parents, understanding the inherent strength their daughter possesses, changed her name again. Among her classmates, she has yet another name—Queen of SIGN Nail.

The orthopaedic surgeons at the hospital who treated Abirah shared that SIGN has a special role in this journey and in giving the message of hope to entire human race. Thank you to ALL SIGN Family.

Boys and Toys

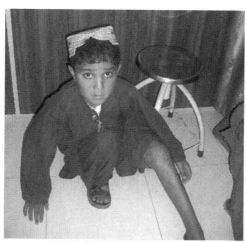

Bashir, a 10-year-old shepherd from Pakistan, was quickly able to return to tending his sheep after SIGN Surgery stabilized his femur.

I was told the following heartwarming story of a Pakistani boy caught in a bomb blast and given a second chance by SIGN Surgeons.

One evening in June 2013, Bashir Ahmad, a 10-year-old shepherd, grazed the family's sheep near his home in *the suburbs of Yaroo, in the Pishin District of Baluchistan, Pakistan. As the sheep foraged, Bashir discovered what he thought was a toy, and he began to play with it as he drove the sheep home.*

A blast sent Bashir's father running to his son. He found the child unconscious with blood-stained clothes and rushed him to the nearby hospital. The doctors there found fractures in both the left humerus (upper arm) and femur (upper leg). They repaired the bones with the methods available to them. An external fixator was placed in the left humerus. An external fixator places pins through the bone connected by a rod and clamps to immobilize the fracture. However, an external fixator limits mobility, and many times the fracture will not heal. Bashir's broken left femur was merely dressed.

Al-Khidmat Al-Hajeri Hospital—or Welfare Trust Hospital—in Quetta, Pakistan, lies over seven hours from Bashir's home in Yaroo; however, it's the closest hospital with orthopaedic surgery facilities. Over one year after the accident in August 2014, Bashir arrived at the Welfare Trust Hospital for treatment. His left femur and left humerus had not healed. The SIGN Surgeons initiated his treatment by removing the external fixator from the humerus and debridement of the wound in the left thigh more than once.

Through SIGN Supporters, who feel the call to help create healing and hope around the world, SIGN is able to provide implants to this program, like many others, at no cost. This enabled the surgeons to repair both Bashir's humerus and femur fractures. It was not long before Bashir was able to return to the business of grazing the family's sheep. He's working now to regain motion in his knee.

According to Bashir's surgeons, the smile on his face gives the message of hope to everyone who sees him!

Simple Gestures Make a Difference

Many humanitarian heroes are recognized at SIGN Conferences. The list is too long to mention them all, but Dr. Pierre Ogedad of Haiti is typical of these heroes.

My experience with SIGN is full of anecdotes, some more exciting than others, but I feel I must share the one that touched me the most.

While doing my daily rounds at Hôpital Sacré Coeur, of Milot, I came across a 50-year-old housewife in the orthopaedic ward. She came to the hospital to have her legs fixed by the visiting orthopaedists. She had been scheduled for surgery, but, unfortunately, it had been canceled the previous day. Seeing her lower limbs, I thought that she was suffering from a limb deformity. I approached her in order to make an examination when I was surprised to see that, far from having a limb deformity, this woman had a nonunion of the lower limbs that had been untreated for about nine months following a fracture of both tibias. Finding it as an interesting case and thinking she might have waited too long, I decided to operate with SIGN Implants in both legs.

The day after the surgery, I went back to review her and see if she could move her lower limbs, and she was able to stand up! Satisfied, I turned to leave the room when I saw her with her arms outstretched to the sky, thanking the Lord for allowing her to stand up again after such a long time. I couldn't imagine that the gesture that I saw as merely surgical was so significant to this woman. I was speechless.

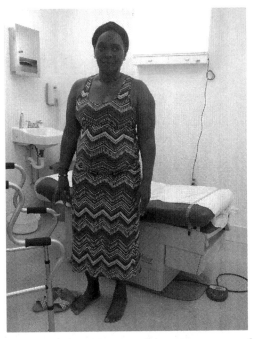

Just one day after SIGN Surgery, this woman was able to stand for the first time since her injury, nine months prior.

Dr. Ogedad's story emphasizes that the involvement of SIGN in Haiti has done more than change the way we perform orthopaedic procedures; SIGN has a great impact on the lives of patients, allowing them to regain the function of their lower extremities and improve their lifestyle. This story helped me to understand that a simple gesture, realized with the ideal and appropriate equipment, could make a huge difference.

Kiwanis—SIGN's Humanitarian Partner

At the 2015 conference, Jeanne Dillner, CEO of all SIGN Operations, applauded one of our great partners.

Kiwanis has been one of SIGN's longest and most reliable partnerships. In 1997, Dr. Lewis Zirkle was named Kiwanis World Service Medal Laureate by the Kiwanis International Foundation. The money received for this award was used to help establish SIGN and cemented a longtime bond between the two organizations. We are proud to announce that Kiwanis has been able to raise more than $1 million for SIGN to treat tens of thousands of patients throughout the world. This year marks the 100th anniversary of the start of Kiwanis. We are incredibly thankful for the support we have received from all Kiwanians. They are always looking for ways to further help the mission of SIGN.

Ann Penner, a member of the Abbotsford Club in British Columbia, Canada, is a perfect example of the lengths Kiwanians will go to help. Ann is the Lt. Governor of the Pacific Northwest District's Division 18 and a member of her District Board. She has been extremely active in Key Club. Under her guidance, her Key Club raised $15,000 to sponsor a SIGN Surgery center in Pakistan. Her dedication to Kiwanis and SIGN seems to have no limits! Ann recently traveled to Cambodia and was kind enough to transport some equipment to the hospitals in need in that region.

At publication, Kiwanis has raised nearly $1.5 million to support SIGN Programs.

Smile of the Week

Dr. Stan Kinsch, a SIGN Surgeon in Kenya, sent this story about a patient with a big smile when he was able to throw away his walking stick.

It is sometimes difficult to find a good start to a newsletter, so let's jump straight into it with a Smile of the Week. This is 54-year-old Peter, who broke his tibia in October 2013. He was treated at the time with plaster casts, but his fracture refused to heal. He was later referred to Coast Provincial Hospital in Mombasa, but he could not afford to buy the plate and nails they wanted to put in his leg. Luckily for him, he then came to Msambweni where I introduced a (free) SIGN Nail in his tibia in January of this year. He is pictured here with a walking stick, but after taking the picture, I told him to lose his walking stick, and he discovered that he could walk without it!

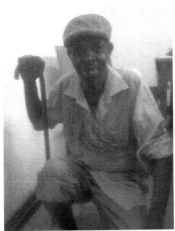

Peter, 54, could not afford the treatment he was first offered when he broke his leg, but a free SIGN Nail helped him heal, walk, and smile.

After I had introduced the general surgeon in Msambweni to those surgeries, he took over a couple of

*my patients and did some very nice SIGN Nails. So that
is, again, a step forward in the sustainability department.*

Paying Kindness Forward

Many surgeons conduct camps in remote areas of their country to
treat the poor who have no access to medical care. Because the SIGN
System is designed to be used in austere environments, these surgeons
can take the equipment where the patients are. Many of these patients
could not afford to travel to the hospital, let alone pay for surgery
and care to heal their injuries. SIGN Surgeons take the SIGN Sets to
conduct camps in Nepal, Tanzania, Somalia, South Sudan, Pakistan,
and many other places. SIGN Surgeons treat all patients with dignity
and skill. Their service is noted during epidemics and disasters, but
humanitarian treatment of the poor occurs on a daily basis.

Dreams Come True

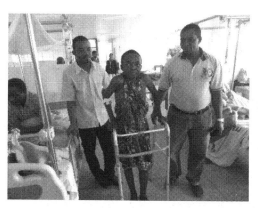

*SIGN Surgery performed by Dr. Billy (right) helped Safiel return to
school within one week of treatment.*

At one of our conferences, Dr. Billy Haonga, chief of the residency program at Muhimbili Orthopaedic Institute in Dar es Salaam.
Tanzania, shared this story about a 15-year-old patient, Safiel Adam.

Safiel is a perfect example of how surgeons like Dr. Billy and our implants can transform a patient's life for the better.

Safiel had just finished primary school and was excited to learn that he passed the test to join secondary education when, just a few days prior to his first day of school, he was involved in a road traffic accident sustaining multiple traumas, including a fracture of the femur. He was taken to a hospital where all of his injuries were treated, except for his broken femur because the hospital did not have the implants needed. As a result, Safiel was put in traction, which failed to heal the fracture. He lay in the ward with his hope of joining his friends in secondary school diminishing more every day.

Dr. Billy met Safiel during an outreach camp visit to the hospital and treated his fracture using a SIGN Implant. "There are no orthopaedic surgeons down there," Dr. Billy said. "We usually travel to their places and operate on them." He was pleased to say how thankful Safiel was to have his leg healed and how hope had been restored by Dr. Billy and SIGN. Safiel was able to return to school the following week to continue to pursue his dreams.

Difficult Fracture Treated in a Mountain Camp

This is a story by Dr. Shazhad Javed of Ghurki Trust Teaching Hospital about Hameeda, whose tibia was healed by a SIGN Nail in an orthopaedic camp in the mountains of Pakistan.

Hameeda Bibi is a 35-year-old woman living in the northern part of Pakistan in the Karakoram Mountains, near the border with China. The Ghurki Trust Teaching Hospital has established an orthopaedic camp there to help with the difficult trauma fractures.

Hameeda broke her tibia when she fell in her home. Following her accident, she visited the local bonesetter, as she had no other immediate facilities to attend to her injury and lacked the funds to travel.

Two weeks after her fall, she found her way to the Ghurki Trust orthopaedic camp and received a SIGN Nail. She was rehabilitated postoperatively and now is able to fully bear weight on her injured leg.

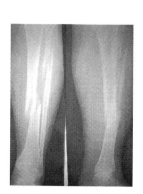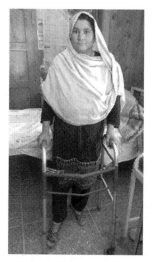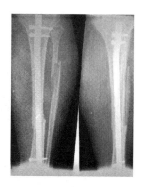

Hameeda, who lives in a remote mountain village, could not afford travel to a hospital, but was able to receive care when SIGN Surgeons held a camp nearby.

Ghurki Trust Teaching Hospital in Lahore, Pakistan, has operated on 2,182 patients using SIGN Implants since the beginning of the SIGN Program in September 2007.

Healing All Ages — the Martha Stories

Jeanne Dillner shared the following two stories from her journey to Tanzania. Coincidentally, each protagonist is named Martha.

Martha the Teenager

I befriended Martha in 2011 when she became the first Tanzanian patient to receive the SIGN Pediatric Nail at Muhimbili Orthopaedic Institute. Martha had been visiting her aunt in Dar es Salaam when she was run over by a group of thieves who were fleeing from the police.

I spent a few days with her as she was recovering from surgery and learned that she was an orphan being raised by her grandmother and that she loved school and wanted to become a teacher. Her surgeon told me that poor families cannot afford to have their children go beyond sixth or seventh grade because of the additional school fees. Seeing that Martha was a bright young girl, I made a commitment to do what I could to enable her to carry out her educational dreams without being a burden to her grandmother.

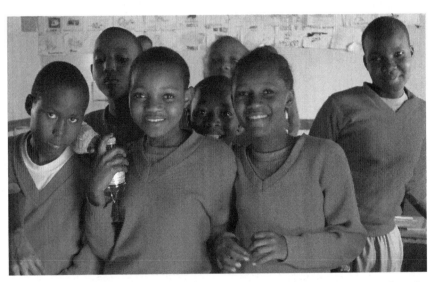

Martha (holding bottle) was the first patient in Tanzania to receive the SIGN Pediatric Nail.

She is now enrolled in a boarding school that's about an hour drive from her grandmother's home, which is located in a village at the base of Mt. Kilimanjaro. She is being taught in Swahili and English. Her English skills enable us to communicate throughout the year, but, as you can imagine, the face-to-face visits are the most rewarding. Now, at 13 years old, Martha is exploring other career options, including engineering. She enjoys math and English and participates fully in net ball, which is a game the girls play every Friday during sports day. During my recent visit, she confirmed that she still loves school. While visiting her classroom, I could tell that she is well-liked by her classmates and is thriving. Seeing her smiling face makes me incredibly thankful to our donors. The gift of SIGN Surgery not only enabled Martha to be healed, but, equally important, allowed her to remain in school to give her a path to a brighter future.

Martha has now changed schools and continues to be sponsored by Jeanne. Dr. Sam Kiwesa, a SIGN Surgeon, and his wife have provided guidance and help for Martha's schooling.

Martha the Matriarch

When I met this Martha, I learned that she had been injured four years prior and left disabled by the untreated fracture to her femur. She did not think surgery was available due to the cost and crawled instead of walking. Undaunted, she crawled around her village to carry out her business and visit friends and family. I envisioned her crawling down dirt roads from houses and shops, each a few feet from each other, similar to the village of the guest house where we were staying.

However, when I joined the hospital driver to take Martha back to her home in the village of Meru, I was surprised that the lovely, one room mud houses, located amidst tall cornstalks and sunflowers, were at least a mile apart. The red clay dirt roads that led to her home were marred with deep crevices caused by the hard rains of recent weeks. I was impressed that neither the distances nor the road conditions nor the inevitable pain she must have endured had deterred this joyful woman from crawling through farm fields and muddy roads for six years to tend her goats, maintain her farm, and visit with her neighbors.

The SIGN Surgery she received enabled her to walk upright again. Martha moves to and from the hospital and through her village surroundings, steadied with the aid of her walker. She continuously thanks her surgeons and SIGN for giving her the surgery that enabled her recovery.

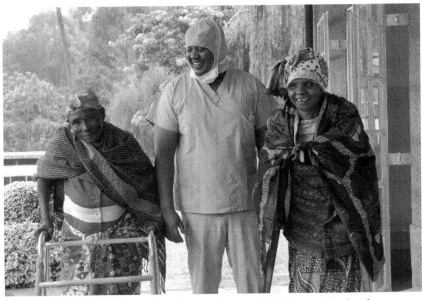

Martha (left) had to crawl in the mud to care for her goats for four years following her injury, until SIGN Surgery enabled her to walk again.

Accident Upsets the Jimba Family

This is a story by Dr. Binod Sherchan, a surgeon at Bir Hospital in Kathmandu, Nepal.

Mrs. Jimba is a 36-year-old female who runs a family of five members including her husband. The family's main source of income comes from a handful of livestock and a sparse patch of land, which only sees crops during one season. Apart from these, Mrs. Jimba and her husband are engaged in daily wage labors. Their combined income barely meets the optimum demand for a standard living.

The life of the Jimba family took an eventful turn-around when Mrs. Jimba was involved in a road traffic accident and sustained a femoral fracture as a passenger in a bus that toppled off the tricky road trail, so often encountered in the mountainous terrain of Nepal. Following the accident, she was brought to Kathmandu, the capital of Nepal, where she sought help in a private hospital, and was managed with an external fixator. The orthopaedic intervention cost the family around 50,000 Nepalese rupees ($800 USD) and her leg was still not healed.

These kinds of cases are frequent occurrences in the only government hospital in a country where people living under the poverty line seek medical support. The hospital services are free, but orthopaedic patients have to procure the implants on their own. A supply of SIGN Implants to these people can be a significant help financially and thus decrease the extra burden on the family's economic capacity, as well as decrease their hospital stay and allow early return to pre-injury functional status.

We strongly believe it would be a great support if

patients in our hospital in Mrs. Jimba's condition could access implants like SIGN Nails. It would be a valuable support to our institution that sees close to 25 orthopaedic surgeries per week.

The SIGN Program was started at Bir Hospital in October 2014.

A Boy's Complicated Journey

This story was written by Dr. Faseeh Shahab, an orthopaedic surgeon in Peshawar, Pakistan.

Treatment which results in timely healing of fractures is expected in the United States. Unfortunately, this is not the case in developing countries. Mohammad is a 12-year-old boy who broke his tibia and femur. He was first treated with traction, but the position of the bones could not be controlled. External fixators were then placed but, again, could not hold the bones in the proper position. A plate was placed on his tibia, as shown on the x-ray. Unfortunately, the plate on the tibia became infected.

When the infection cleared, flexible nails were placed into the femur to hold reduction. These nails were removed, but the patient's femur still had not healed.

After 13 months of despair and failed treatments at hospitals in a neighboring country, Mohammad's parents took him to Lady Reading Hospital in Peshawar, Pakistan, where he was treated with a SIGN Nail. We attribute his successful healing to the SIGN Surgeons at this hospital.

We are deeply grateful to dedicated supporters who make it possible for us to continue to supply SIGN Surgeons with what Pakistani surgeons affectionately call the "Magic Nail." They call it the "Magic Nail" because the results are so good when it is used in their patients. I believe most of the "magic" is because the surgeons are so good. Pakistan surgeons have used SIGN Implants to heal nearly 10,000 patients since we started SIGN after the earthquake in 2007.

Realities of Life

Dr. Rizwan Akram, a surgeon in Pakistan, wrote this story about a milkman who was detained from his deliveries.

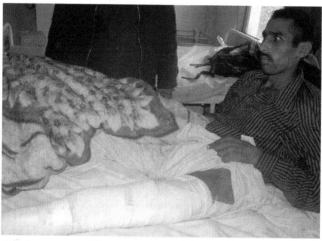

Ghulam was able to return to his work as a milkman thanks to a successful SIGN Surgery.

Ghulam Hur is a 25-year-old male living in Pakistan. He earns a living by working as a milkman. In December, he was involved in a road traffic accident while delivering milk. He sustained injuries to his head and left thigh and was taken to a hospital in Lahore, Pakistan, for treatment. Several of Ghulam's injuries were operated on by the department of neurosurgery. He was then put on a ventilator for 15 days. To resolve his fractured femur, he was put in skin traction and lay in bed for 45 days. He lost *approximately 50,000 rupees ($930 USD) of his earnings due to missing work and the expense of treatment.*

Ghulam could not afford further treatment, but he had heard about a nearby SIGN Program at Ghurki Trust Teaching Hospital. He was admitted, and after six days of skeletal traction he received his SIGN Surgery. Ghulam is recovering and improving greatly each day. Thank you, SIGN, for helping our poor and deserving patients. These are not just stories about patients—they are realities of life.

Surgeon Returns Home

Dr. Akau Aguto, an orthopaedic surgeon, returned to South Sudan to Juba Teaching Hospital to provide fracture care to his countrymen recovering from the devastation of war.

South Sudan is the newest member of the United Nations after independence from Sudan on July 9, 2011. The land and people suffered tremendously from a civil war that lasted almost 50 years. The little infrastructure the country had was destroyed during the civil war. South Sudan has a population of about 10 million distributed in 10 states. There has been no functioning fracture care in all of South Sudan, partially due to lack of facilities and/or absence of an orthopaedic surgeon. Trauma patients are referred from 10 states to the capital city, Juba, with the hope of finding appropriate fracture care in the center.

The Department of Orthopaedics has 46 beds and triple that amount of patients, who use the floor as beds. Juba Teaching Hospital (JTH) offers only skeletal traction to treat many cases of fracture shaft femur. This means these patients occupy hospital beds for six weeks. No surprise that JTH has high incidence of all complications related to long hospital stays with patients lying in skeletal traction. Bed sores, respiratory infections, urinary tract infections, DVT and traumatic osteomyelitis are a few examples of the many complications experienced.

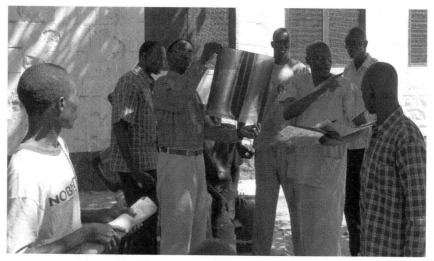

Dr. Akau (right, pointing) returned to his homeland as soon as South Sudan gained independence in 2011. He is one of the only orthopaedic surgeons in the country.

Now with me being originally from South Sudan and a Norwegian-trained orthopaedic surgeon (also Norwegian citizen), I felt obliged to move back to South Sudan with a hope of making a difference in fracture care, traumatology and orthopaedics. I had a privilege of learning the SIGN System in Malawi under supervision of a friend and colleague, Dr. Sven Young.

I am looking forward with much anticipation to make a revolution in fracture care in South Sudan should the SIGN Family add Juba Teaching Hospital to its membership. SIGN Fellowship will benefit the 10 million who live in South Sudan.

The SIGN Program started at Juba Teaching Hospital in July 2012, and 639 patients have been treated using SIGN Implants.

Waiting for the Rooster

Henry Ndasi, a surgeon at Baptist Hospital Mutengene in Cameroon, wanted very much to provide proper care for his patients. He explains the difficulty in this story.

It is common knowledge that over time a fracture will heal in some form, regardless of any intervention. In Cameroon, Africa, if a patient has a fractured leg they go to a "bone doctor." These "doctors" use a local custom of catching a rooster, fracturing one of its legs and waiting for it to heal. Once the rooster can walk again, it is assumed the patient should be healed as well. Unfortunately, due to a shortage of trained orthopaedic surgeons in Cameroon, many people rely on this type of treatment. Even if patients do go see a trained doctor, they often cannot afford treatment.

It is within this setting that I am starting my ortho-paedic practice. I am the only trained orthopaedist in the area. Baptist Hospital Mutengene, where I am start-ing my practice, currently has 60 beds which are filled to 100–110% occupancy. Since this is a faith-based non-profit hospital, we do not turn down treatment for anyone who is sick. The problem is many patients cannot afford to pay their medical bills, and therefore we struggle to break even and keep the hospital afloat.

This explains why starting a practice in the midst of real need has been difficult. In anticipation of my orthopaedic practice, plans had been made to build a new surgical suite and wards. Unfortunately, the finances could not be raised. Instead, we modified parts of the current wards, transforming them into two operating rooms.

I have an average of five cases a day. If emergency surgeries arise, we tend to run out of recyclable surgical gowns. If we do too many surgeries on consecutive days, our small laundry machines cannot cope with the load, leaving us without adequate gowns to operate in. We cannot afford to provide food to our patients, and at times this causes a bit of a crisis. One asks whether we are to provide treatment to this patient or something as basic as food.

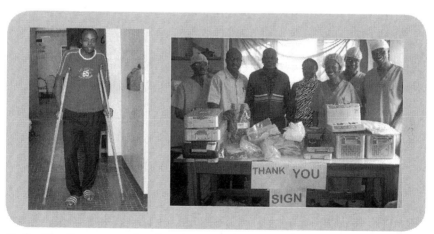

Left: Abraham was the first patient at Baptist Hospital Mutengene to receive SIGN Surgery, and he was quickly able to walk and return to work.

Right: The team from Baptist Hospital Mutengene in Cameroon celebrated when they received their SIGN Set.

Despite these difficult circumstances, not all patients are full of misery. Baptist Hospital Mutengene received its SIGN System in March, and I was able to do my first SIGN

Surgery a few weeks later. My first patient, Abraham, a 32-year-old motorcyclist, was involved in a road traffic accident. He lay in bed waiting for three weeks for the SIGN System to reach our hospital. Abraham and his wife were very happy he could have his fracture fixed for free. He was back on his feet within a couple of days of surgery and soon returned to work.

The SIGN Program started in Baptist Hospital Mutengene in Cameroon in March 2012, and 499 surgeries have been performed using SIGN Implants. Dr. Henry wants to build a trauma center to more efficiently care for the many trauma patients he sees.

Filipino Surgeon Almost Gives Up

Trained at Southern Philippines Medical Center and now practicing in the Philippines, Dr. Luigi "Gio" Andrew Sabal describes horrendous conditions and how SIGN helped and restored his desire to practice in his homeland.

There is a hole in my bed—big enough that if you move right over it, you might fall through. My water has been out for two years, so every day I spend an hour fetching water in a pail just so that me and my wife can bathe. I earn about $400 a month. Tough huh? That's life from my side of the world.

I'm not a patient; I am a doctor in the Philippines. By most standards here, I am living a pretty good life. The same cannot be said for the people I serve. My patients are poor. It is ironic that the men and women who work longer and harder than me earn less than me, but the majority of our patients earn less than a dollar or two a day and have no savings whatsoever. I'm like you in many ways, except that I get paid in fruits, crabs, and live chickens. I work in a government training institution in the Southern Philippines. We're no strangers to motor vehicular accidents that break almost every imaginable bone in the body. I see horrible mangled extremities from casualties of war, and falls from coconut trees that can shatter a person's spine. All in a day's work where I'm from.

The operating rooms I work in lack the standard "basic" surgical equipment, and the air conditioning seldom works. We only have two lead gowns for the entire staff, so 12 residents share the same gowns, while the nurses go out of the rooms whenever we operate with fluoroscopy. But we're lucky. A few years ago our institution didn't have lead gowns. When one of our graduates passed away, it was rumored to be caused by the radiation exposure in the operating room.

The emergency supplies are limited to betadine and gauze, so when patients come in the emergency room we are forced to send them out again to buy the necessary supplies. Let's say a guy walks in with a broken leg accompanied by his mother. We put him on a bed, write out a prescription and send his mother out again into the night to buy the casting materials. But what if the said guy doesn't have money or needs more than just casting materials? Things like anesthesia, sutures, antibiotics, and IV fluids still have to be bought in pharmacies outside the emergency room. What then?

If I had some cash on me, I'd be able to buy supplies for my patient. For a time I tried that, but it was a habit I could not afford. The government helps to pay to some extent, but not entirely. So we (the residents) pool our resources and make sure that nothing goes to waste.

As an orthopaedic surgeon, the largest bulk of the financial expense would be that of the implants. Since the Philippines do not manufacture orthopaedic implants, most of the implants are imported from other parts of Asia. Unfortunately, the affordable ones are of questionable quality. But as an orthopaedic training institution, we are lucky; we have a long-term collaboration with SIGN.

Over the past 10 years, with the help of the SIGN Nail, the average length of a hospital stay has been cut from 23 days to 12 days at present. The SIGN Nail is a versatile tool we use for most fractures of the femur and tibia. Thanks to its ease of use and design, intraoperative imaging is not necessary.

There was a time when I was working in a hospital that did not have an active SIGN Program. Patients were in traction for weeks due to their inability to pay for the necessary implants. I remember crying outside the ward because I felt so helpless for my patients. It was as if whatever I did, did not matter, that I did not matter. The feeling was so depressing that I questioned my role as a surgeon and left my profession for six months.

During my leave I contemplated working abroad. I wanted to focus on treating my patients and not worrying about where to find money so that they could receive treatment. What could an individual do? Back then logging on to social networks only made things worse when I looked up medical school classmates who were working in developed countries. They were earning 10 times more than doctors here, not worrying about where to find their patient's medicines and surgical requirements.

But if I left, who would take care of the patients here?

In the end I decided not to leave; better to serve in my home country. That was when I transferred to my current training institution, Southern Philippines Medical Center. SIGN has helped patients, no question about that, but they have also helped doctors. Through the SIGN Program young doctors, such as myself, have been given the opportunity to train in orthopaedic trauma without worrying if our patients could afford to purchase the implants. SIGN is concerned about each and every patient.

We, as residents, send pre- and post-operative x-rays to the SIGN Database. Not only do we learn technique and management strategies from our local experience, but we also learn from the cases done in other parts of the world. SIGN has opened the doors for us to the world. People whose names we only read in books are corresponding with us and sharing their ideas through SIGN. I've been to orthopaedic conventions around the world, but nothing compares to the annual SIGN Conference. The environment is so warm and friendly. Initially, I felt insecure that I came from a developing country with limited resources. I felt I had nothing to contribute to first world orthopaedic surgeons. But it was a pleasant surprise that even our little ideas, like mini-open incision reductions for fracture reduction or various entry points in the greater trochanter, were received with enthusiasm and appreciation.

SIGN restored my belief that there was something I could do for my country in my own way. That I didn't have to leave the country to make a difference; that I still mattered.

I am not a patient, I am a doctor, and thanks to SIGN, I can help my country without leaving. So, with that being said, will YOU help SIGN?

Unsung Heroes in Haiti

Jeanne Dillner reports on building orthopaedic capacity in the wake of disaster, in this case, the 2010 earthquake in Haiti.

Every overseas trip reveals something new about the SIGN Surgeons, SIGN as an organization, and about myself. The first impression I want to convey is the strength and perseverance of the orthopaedic residents in Haiti. These individuals lost colleagues, friends, family, and in many cases their facilities; yet they continue to treat the barrage of humanity streaming into their makeshift wards and surgical suites. Dr. Gilbert Gourdet showed us a database of the cases they performed during and since the earthquake. They knew they would be caring for these patients long-term and wanted to record these cases and obtain follow-ups to confirm that patients were getting good results.

Twelve residents from Haiti University and Education Hospital attended the 2010 SIGN Conference. Their demeanor reflected the emotional trauma they experienced during the aftermath of the quake, so it was difficult to tell whether they were benefiting from the courses. One goal we had for this conference was to see how SIGN Training was being implemented in their hospital.

Tuesday morning one lecture hall was transformed into a Ponseti clinic. The Ponseti method is a non-surgical

168

method of treating children born with clubfoot. Chief resident Dr. Chertoute Getho told us they started these clinics after completing the Ponseti workshop at the SIGN Conference.

The same morning, fourth year resident Dr. Eldine Jacques was showing Dr. Zirkle the flap cases she had performed. Flaps are used by plastic surgeons to repair soft tissue damage. Orthopaedic surgeons in developing countries rarely have access to plastic surgeons, so they must learn this technique. University of California San Francisco held a flap course workshop two days prior to the SIGN Conference where SIGN Surgeons could practice on cadavers. Dr. Eldine was not able to attend, but she learned how to do flaps from a thumb drive of the course material that was distributed at the SIGN Conference.

We were further impressed by the caliber of surgery that was being performed. Dr. Zirkle scrubbed in on some very difficult cases. I noticed that the residents were scrubbing in and performing the duties of orthopaedic nurses. Drs. Gilbert and Getho had mentioned earlier their frustration at having to organize and prepare the instruments and implants for sterilization, and that they also had to perform scrub nurse duties. This is a typical scene in many developing countries, and I agreed with them that they needed a training program for the nurses and surgical technicians; however, the tragedy of their need did not resonate with me until Dr. Mukkuaka Oda gave me a tour of the hospital grounds. We walked by the general surgery wing, which is now condemned and will be torn down, and the orthopaedic surgical wing, which was already torn down. That's when it sunk in that orthopaedic surgeons are vying with general surgeons for the limited time available in the operating suites. The orthopaedic wards are crowded because there are not enough operating rooms available.

As we talked, an email we received from Dr. Francel Alexis the day after the quake crept into my memory. He said, "It is horrible, the nurses' college is flattened. We've lost everybody." I remember the impact that email had on me a year ago, and I was embarrassed and frustrated with myself that it took this long for me to recall that message. As we walked by the residents' living quarters, Dr. Oda said, "See that tree? Before the earthquake, the nursing college was in the foreground and we never saw that tree. That day we lost 200 nurses, teachers and our colleagues." Behind the nursing college was the medical college which also fell to the ground and where they lost another 200 students and professors. That tree is a heartbreaking reminder of the loss. I equate their view to that of New Yorkers who no longer see the Twin Towers. These young men and women who survived, worked under a cloud of dust and grief to treat the living while they mourned their lost. I hope you join me in acclaiming the Haitian surgeons and medical personnel as the unsung heroes of the 2010 earthquake.

SIGN Programs Taking Root

Volunteer surgeon Dr. Carla Smith, who also serves on the SIGN Board of Directors, reflects on her visit to Nepal.

As I boarded the Thai Airways Flight from Los Angeles International Airport to Bangkok on my ninth trip to Nepal, the eighth trip for SIGN, I realized that

I was living my dream. The anxiety and unknown that was so exhilarating on that first trip had been replaced with a relative contentment that however the trip evolved, it would be as it should.

Several previous times I had tried to travel within Nepal to visit remote hospitals where SIGN had been initiated by surgeons who traveled to Kathmandu to learn the procedure. Many times the political unrest and the countermeasures taken by the government to restrict the Maoist uprisings had thwarted travel and paralyzed the country, causing a cessation of road traffic and domestic flights.

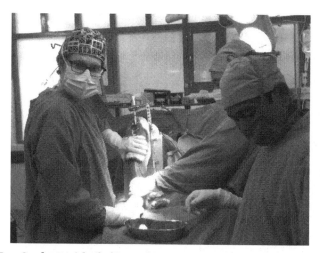

Dr. Carla Smith (left) performs SIGN Surgery in Nepal.

This was to be my first trip to the mission hospital in Tansen, a village perched on the mountainside between Pokhara and the Indian border to the south. One of the Kathmandu SIGN Surgeons and his university friend, an ardent supporter of the emerging tourist homestay travel program in the region, escorted me. As I successfully passed customs with my carefully packed 110 pounds of medical equipment and my two outfits, including my puffy orange down coat, I entered the bright daylight of a clear winter day and encountered the ever-enthusiastic Dr. Chakra Pandey, my first SIGN Surgeon contact and now a close family friend.

His vision for a regional trauma referral center in Kathmandu is as bold and audacious as Lew Zirkle's vision of an implant which equalizes fracture care throughout the world and equally likely, given the drive and talent backing it. One-third completed, it may be the first facility to realize function as a regional training center for SIGN. Seeing the progress over the last eight months since my previous visit confirmed the commitment to this project.

Spending the following day with Chakra's children confirmed the effect he is having on those around him. His eldest daughter is poised to leave the nest and intends to do so in dramatic fashion, intending to pursue international relations with an emphasis on the role of women in emerging societies. Though quiet and studious, she has clearly assimilated Chakra's values.

The following day was spent in transit to Tansen from Kathmandu, an arduous journey for the drivers— my surgeon colleague, Suman, and his friend, Navin. I was happily oblivious to the oncoming traffic and near-miss reality of the nine-hour drive, happily tucked in the back seat with my electronic books, happy for a moment of quiet from my normal work existence. We were amply filled with milk, tea, and daal bhat [steamed rice and lentil soup] en route and arrived safely at the family home of Navin, high atop the ridge above Tansen. His family warmly greeted us with hot tea and dinner, cooked in the dark over gas stoves due to the load-sharing blackouts still ever-present in Nepal.

Tansen Mission Hospital is a decades-old hospital tucked in the hillside at Tansen, now staffed by Dr. Dipak, who, with the help of one senior and one junior resident, mans the busy trauma service. I assisted Dr. Subin, the senior resident, with a tibial nail first case in the morning and was very impressed with his technical skills and ability, and especially his respect for his instruments. Following that, we all (Dipak, Subin, Suman, and I) scrubbed for a femoral head fracture/dislocation. Through a Smith–Peterson approach, we placed two 2.7 screws and appreciated the stability that engendered for the infra-foveal fracture. We followed with a tibial plateau fracture and managed to have time to review research cases and x-rays and still make it to an early dinner together.

I was most impressed by the dedication, commit-ment, and energy that Drs. Dipak and Subin dedicate to their patients. Tansen is very efficient and well run, and operating there very enjoyable. I look forward to hearing Subin's full presentation at the next SIGN Conference, having reviewed their experience with the timing of operative repair of pediatric supracondylar humeral fractures.

Returning safely to Kathmandu, I was able to spend a full operating day at Patan Hospital, two years into its SIGN Program, and performed two SIGN Nails, one decep-tively easy and the other irritatingly elusive. Both were closed without difficulty, and a number of other cases were performed as well. From there, I revisited Nepal Medical College briefly, one of the oldest programs in the country, and then on to *Nepal Orthopaedic Hospital, by far the busiest orthopaedic hospital in the SIGN Program in Nepal.*

One of the benefits of repeated visits is the network of friends that I now count in Nepal. A day did not go by without tea or daal with friends, and the number of invitations easily outnumbered the evenings of the trip. Each visit now deepens my realization that there will always be another trip and another chance to renew acquaintances. The energy of novelty has matured into the calm of knowing that SIGN is in the capable hands of devoted surgeons and that new programs will spring from existing programs. I am now merely the water that sustains the programs; the roots are sown and the seeds will spread.

Return to the Scene of the Crime

Dr. Kyle Dickson tells of his return to Muhimbili Orthopaedic Institute in Dar es Salaam, Tanzania. Dickson, from Houston, TX, is an internationally known orthopaedic surgeon who makes one trip per year to SIGN Programs. His teaching is treasured by SIGN Surgeons.

Some have suggested that fixing chronic pelvic and acetabular malunions and nonunions with iliosacral screws in a third world country without a C-arm is a crime. People usually tell me, "You are either crazy or insane." I then tell them about the patients who were previously unable to walk for six months and now are able to return to work and reply, "No, the real crime is how much waste is in our own health care system and how much the Muhimbili Orthopaedic Institute in combination with SIGN can do with so little."

In my experience, the giver of charity has a much more profound experience than the receiver. My second trip to Dar es Salaam was no exception. Besides the wonderful swims in the Indian Ocean alongside beautiful beaches, the cultural richness of the National Museum of Tanzania, and the breathtaking safaris of Ngorongoro Crater, Dar es Salaam offers a surgeon a greater appreciation for what he or she has back home, as well as the power of the human spirit to accomplish what most would think impossible. As Cardinal Suewens says, "Happy are those who dream and are willing to pay the price to make those dreams come true."

I arrived on Saturday night and visited the National Museum of Tanzania on Sunday. The country is somewhat unique in Africa in its relatively quiet self-governance. Problems still exist, i.e. all the big houses are owned by government workers, but the industry of the people both at the harbor and in the hospital are truly remarkable.

As was the case last year, there were too many cases with not enough hours in a day to finish them all. Due to the extreme poverty and great distances, we operatively treated numerous acetabular and pelvic injuries that were over two months old with the hip still dislocated and femoral head fractured. The cases went great, the patients were so appreciative, and the staff and doctors at Muhimbili Orthopaedic Institute (MOI) treated me like I was a rock star. The dedicated doctors at Muhimbili were significantly more advanced than their already high level of sophistication the previous year.

I gave three lectures in a standing-room-only conference classroom on Plafond Fractures, Disaster or Success?, Femoral Neck Fractures, To Fix or Replace, *and Pelvic and Acetabular Malunions and Nonunions: The Good, The Bad, and The Ugly. We had a thought-provoking discussion, and their level of expertise was impressive. They had excellent questions and an unquenchable thirst for knowledge. Clearly with the SIGN Program, they have come a long way and are dedicated to improvement and perfection. Experience is not doing a better job for the patient, but doing a perfect job more efficiently.*

Lest you think I'm a workaholic, I did spend the last two days on a safari in the Ngorongoro Crater and at Lake Victoria. As I watched a lioness less than five feet from me returning from a kill covered in blood, I could not help but feel a symbiosis with this big cat, the environment, and the Tanzanian people. So many countries in Africa are constantly in turmoil. Tanzania has succeeded in preserving the environment and wildlife with co-habitation with humans, i.e. the Maasai tribe. This cooperation is similar to the relationship between the Muhimbili Orthopaedic Institute, SIGN, and the injured people of Tanzania. Risk, more than others think, is safe. Care, more than others think, is wise. Dream, more than others think, is practical. Expect more than others think is possible. Add all these together and you have Tanzania.

Nurse Becomes a Patient

The woman pictured below is a ward nurse at Mitford Hospital in Dhaka, Bangladesh. This hospital serves the district where the majority of the rickshaw drivers live. The SIGN Program was started here by Dr. Faruque Quasem. This nurse knows how fractures used to be treated before the SIGN Program began. She knows that the poorest of the poor remained bedridden for months because the hospital did not have access to free implants to treat their badly fractured legs. In contrast, when she was hit by a car, she was taken into surgery within two hours to receive a SIGN Nail, and now rests comfortably in the ward, knowing that she can return home soon and that her leg will return to its full function. Thanks to the persistence and quality of surgeries by Dr. Faruque and his team, the rickshaw drivers and others from the poorest district in Dhaka can now receive equal orthopaedic care.

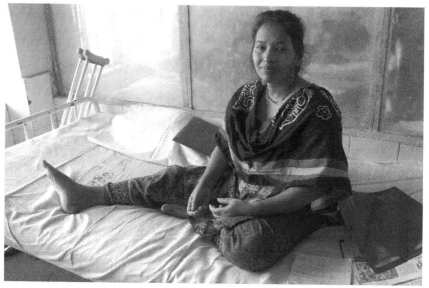

This nurse can smile because she knows that she has received the best treatment for her broken leg—a SIGN Nail.

Dr. Faruque started the SIGN Program at National Institute of Traumatology and Orthopedic Rehabilitation Hospital (NITOR) in Dhaka, Bangladesh, in September 2002, and 1,326 SIGN Surgeries have been done there. Dr. Faruque moved to Sir Salimullah Medical College (SSMC) Mitford Hospital in Dhaka in 2010 where his team has done 333 SIGN Surgeries since inception of the program.

A Healing Chain

Dr. Aung Thein Htay of Yangon General Hospital in Myanmar tells this story about the united effort of surgeons, equipment provider, and family to heal the patient.

Win Htein is a 43-year-old truck mechanic from Thone Gwa Township in Myanmar. One day while working, he fell from one of the trucks, breaking his left femur. Win's family of six was shaken when their breadwinner was bedridden. They depended on the $6 a day that he brought home to support them. Win was taken to Yangon General Hospital to get treatment, but, unfortunately, a shortage of blood in the hospital delayed his surgery. Win's caring wife volunteered to donate her blood so that her husband could get the treatment he so badly needed, and it just so happened she matched his blood type.

The surgeons got right to work donating their time and a SIGN Implant to get Win back on his feet. After the operation, Win's wife was there waiting for him, proudly wearing a T-shirt given to her by the National Blood Bank for her donation.

It took the kindness of many people to help Win regain his health. The blood from his wife, the time from the surgeons, and a SIGN Implant created a healing chain of giving to restore Win and get him back to work.

Dr. Aung has assumed the leadership of the SIGN Programs in Myanmar, led by the Yangon General Hospital. He teaches the new SIGN Surgeons in Myanmar and has personally started many SIGN Programs. Yangon General Hospital has performed 3,552 SIGN Surgeries since the program began.

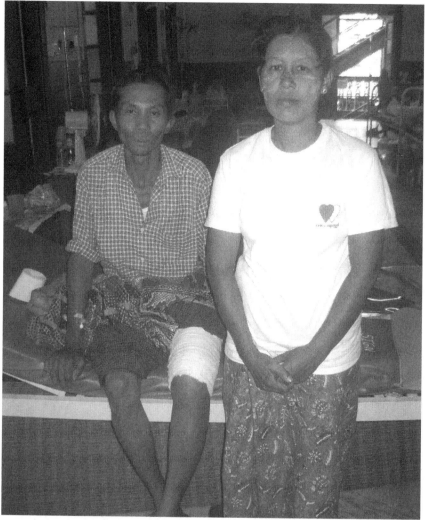

This man (left) was healed thanks to the care of SIGN Surgeons and blood donated by his wife (right).

Life-Saving Surgery

Dr. Mansoor Ilyas of Sajid Hospital in Quetta, Pakistan, treated a patient whose motorcycle ran over a mine.

Quetta is the capital city of the province of Balochistan, which has been wasted by an armed insurgence the past 10 years. In the midst of conflict, everyday people are struggling to work and raise their children.

Raees, a father of seven children, ran over a mine with his motor-cycle while he was delivering his buffalo milk to buyers in Sibi City. Raees' injuries were life threatening. He suffered a shrapnel puncture to his left femoral artery. Fortunately, his attendant knew there was a doctor in Quetta, 100 kilometers away, who had the instruments and the training to treat him properly. That orthopaedic surgeon was Dr. Mansoor.

After several transfers, Raees was brought to Dr. Mansoor at Sajid Hospital. Within a matter of 48 hours, the metal was removed from Raees' left leg, the exposed bone was covered, and in one sitting all the fractures were fixed with the SIGN System. The next morning Raees was able to sit with one leg on the chair. The operation was a success by US standards and a lifesaver by Balochi standards.

Dr. Mansoor finished his triumphant report with this humbling sentiment: "In our country the poor do not have a future. Through your help, we save families from starvation and disaster for which all family members are so thankful."

Boosts Confidence

The 2016 SIGN Conference boosted the confidence of Dr. Emal Yaqubi from Afghanistan.

SIGN Conferences and other trainings facilitated through SIGN are not only improving technical skills, but are inspiring and motivating venues for young surgeons like me. Every time I return to my country, I go with tons of applicable ideas which are affordable and sustainable in my setting to improve patient care. In the meantime, attending the conferences boosts confidence in my own technical expertise by comparing my patient care with other developing countries. I love the SIGN slogan to provide equal fracture care around the world because SIGN provides the same intramedullary nail to everybody worldwide, no matter how rich or poor is the individual.

With the support of SIGN, I can now fix fractures (with a less invasive approach) and can do skin grafts if needed, as Afghan surgeons deal a lot with gunshot injuries. I can also consult on some complicated cases with SIGN Surgeons to provide quality treatment for my patients and use their lessons learned. SIGN facilitated for me to observe sports medicine surgeries in US, which was a very good experience, and I have already started to motivate investors to invest in arthroscopic surgery equipment to provide less invasive and more effective surgical treatment in the country.

Changed Concepts

At the 2016 SIGN Conference, Dr. Shazhad Javed of Ghurki Trust Teaching Hospital in Pakistan took a workshop that benefited his colleagues and patients.

This training was very suitable and good for me because the only thing weak at our center was pelvis fracture treatment, and after attending the workshop we have now started performing a lot of fixation here and helping poor patients—especially with post wall fracture anterior open book fracture, closed external fixator, anterior screw, and plates for SI joints. This training helped us and changed our concepts. We need this event every year to learn more and more. Thanks for such a good workshop.

New Ideas

The 2016 SIGN Conference gave new ideas and sharpened skills to Dr. Akimu Mageza of Parirenyatwa Hospital in Zimbabwe.

I was very honored to be a delegate for the September 2016 training, and my appreciation also extends to the donors for making it possible for us to travel and partici-pate in such a great training.

The training improved my skills in management of fractures through discussions, exchanges and the con-ference in Richland. New ideas were brought up and attained through exchanging information and this will go a long way as I continue in the practice. In Seattle, we learnt largely about the management of pelvic and spine injuries. This was very helpful and insightful as it improved our understanding of the topic and the man-agement thereof.

The conference and trainings brought new ideas, which improved my skills, helped my practice, and sharp-ened my skills. Also, when I got back, I managed to share the new ideas and learnings with my colleagues so as to help improve locally in our communities.

No Man's Land No More

Dr. Jacky Jean of Haiti is helping his fellow surgeons believe that they can treat complex injuries, thanks to SIGN's efforts.

Dear friends,

Thank you is not really enough to say to every single person that donated either their time or their money to make this happen. Without your help, it would have been

182

difficult, even impossible for me to make it.

Your efforts are changing and will continue to change people's lives after decades. I believe. Before, in my country the trend was: "Do not touch the pelvis," "Do not touch the acetabulum," "Do not touch the spine." No man's land. Now, even little by little, I've started to make them believe if everybody in the world is doing those kind of surgeries, so can we.

Imagine this 43-year-old lady, this 25-year-old man and this 30-year-old man would have become crippled, with chronic pain, without the surgery for their pelvic and acetabular fractures.

Thank you one more time and please continue to help others with your priceless efforts, so that we would become a better place.

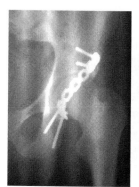 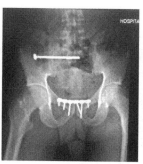 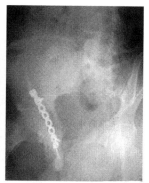

Dr. Jacky Jean sent these x-rays to illustrate the surgeries.

Trimodal Benefit

I am Dr. Ijaz Ahmad working as a consultant orthopaedic and spine surgeon at Ghurki Trust Teaching Hospital in Lahore, Pakistan. I got introduced to SIGN in 2004, courtesy of Dr. Ajmal Yasin, my teacher at medical school and himself a practicing orthopaedic surgeon.

Since then we have been doing SIGN Nailing for fractures of humerus, femur, and tibia. We have done more than 1,000 cases to date with a reasonably good follow-up. I was proud to be a part of 2011 and 2013 SIGN Conferences, where I had the honor of presenting my papers as well.

SIGN has been a great blessing for my patients and hospital. Pakistan is a LMIC (low and middle income country). We have a poor health infrastructure with a very poor per capita income. There is no health insurance system, and patients have to spend for their treatment from their own pockets. That's why many non-affording patients do not even report to hospitals when they fall ill or get fractures. In this gloomy background, SIGN emerged as a ray of hope and light for these poor and needy. Patients started getting quality implants free of cost, and hospitals started bearing the burden of medicine for most of them. We generated a ward fund based on donations from different local donors and arranged for medication and rehabilitation of the patients receiving SIGN Nails. SIGN really changed the horizon of adult long bone fracture management in our hospital. In my opinion, SIGN has been a source of trimodal benefit for us.

Patients get solid intra-medullary implants free of cost. Most patients returned to their pre-injury ambulatory status and jobs after SIGN Surgeries. This brought happiness in many families as most male patients were sole bread-earners of their families.

Hospital patient turnover increased. Satisfied patients boosted the confidence of the common man in our hospital and health system.

Consultants and trainees got more operating opportunities which resulted in better training of future orthopaedic surgeons.

Last, but not the least, I have to thank Dr. Lewis Zirkle and his whole team for being a great help for ailing humanity across the globe.

No More Tough Times

Dr. Mohammad Moazzam Ghori with his colleague Dr. Latifur Rehman describes his accidental discovery of SIGN and the difference it has made in Quetta, Pakistan.

My story starts five years back when I traveled to visit my sister in Abbottabad in the Khyber Pakhtunkhwa state of Pakistan.

A neighboring patient with a frozen shoulder wanted help. I asked a local hospital to do manipulation under anesthesia of the patient, and they allowed me to use their operation theater. After doing the procedure on my way out, I saw a patient waiting with SIGN Nail x-rays in her hand which I never seen before. She was looking for the surgeon to take the SIGN Nail out after her fracture was cured. In meantime, the surgeon came, and after intro-duction, my first question was about the SIGN Nail. I was surprised to know that it can be passed without using image, and the surgeon gave me the contact information for SIGN. The surgeon was Dr. Ali Asghar Shah.

On my return back home to Al Khidmet Al Hajeri Hospital in Quetta, we started to contact SIGN, and in the middle of correspondence, the coordinator, Mr. Sultan, left the job and proceeded to Afghanistan for good.

There was a gap in contact when an orthopaedic surgeons' conference was held in Quetta and some funds were generated. This time I introduced Dr. Mansoor Ilyas to SIGN and we opened an office in Sajid Hospital and hired a coordinator to contact SIGN. We were fortunate to start the SIGN Program in Sajid Hospital.

After some time, a new doctor, Dr. Latifur Rahman, joined Al Khidmet Hospital and I informed him about SIGN and we were again fortunate to start the program at Al Khidmet Hospital in Quetta, Pakistan.

SIGN changed the direction of fracture cure in the area where nearly all the patients treated with locally made equipment were returning with broken nails, lose or broken screws, and the condition which nobody wants to see—severe infection. Now, for the patient, it is one-day admission, the next day surgery, and the third day go home and play soccer!

The operating theater staff now has time for breaks. They are very comfortable with the easy introduction of SIGN Nails and smooth surgeries. Nobody has seen the tough times like before.

Myself, I have the chance to sleep now comfortably in the night and, also, can even have a nap at noon, if I'm not seeing any complicated case.

SIGN Inspires a Career

Dr. Sami Hailu of Ethiopia describes his SIGN Journey.

Unlike many SIGN Surgeons, I got introduced to SIGN in time of need. It was just three weeks after I graduated from medical school, when I was involved in motor vehicle accident and broke my right thigh bone (femur) in two different places (segmental fracture). The first thing that came to my mind when I realized I broke my femur was three months of skeletal traction in a Perkins bed. I couldn't think of anything else, because that was what I'd seen in medical school while in training—rows of Perkins beds with femur fractures on skeletal traction. SIGN was not introduced to my hospital at that time.

The accident happened 250 kilometers away from Addis Ababa, where the best centers in the country are available (at least to my understanding at that time). So I had to be transported in a minibus to Addis. The first aid that we get for traumas in Ethiopia in general are way below the standard. In my case, an intern in Hawassa Referral Hospital put me on long leg posterior gutter which was short of the proximal fracture site. We drove in the public transport minibus to Addis with me in pain and arrived there after midnight. I believe that was the worst car ride I can ever imagine in my life, and for that I will never forget the night's six-hour ride from the southern part of Ethiopia to Addis.

I was put on skin traction, got some analgesic, and got admitted to hospital. It was during this moment I was introduced to SIGN, when I asked what the options were to manage my fracture. For different reasons, that I don't want to mention here, I waited for 16 days on skin traction till I got my fractures fixed with a SIGN Nail. Mind you, I waited this long with broken bones and I was a physician. I think it is not difficult to imagine about the fate of my poor countrymen who suffer similar and even worse injuries in Ethiopia, who have no idea or means on *how to get to these centers when they break their bones. Time and a new generation of hard-working people will change this beyond doubt, but that is what the reality is for most us here in Ethiopia.*

With this experience, I couldn't think of specializing in anything else other than to become an orthopod. Literally speaking, SIGN made me join the orthopaedics training program six months right after my accident. That is when I realized that SIGN has changed the whole practice of orthopaedics in the department from what I knew while in medical school. No more rows of patients in Perkins traction, no more three months of hospital bed occupancy for femur fractures. It is indeed gratifying to see fractures fixed and the patient discharged in few days after the injury. This, to my mind, is the way forward in fracture care.

I don't want to be misquoted here though. I am not saying things have totally changed. But I see a bright future in fracture care, even though we have got a lot to do in improving the efficiency of managing these injuries and improve the standard of more complex trauma management (like open injuries, periarticular fractures, pelvic and acetabulum). A talented young generation of orthopaedic surgeons is being trained and graduating, thanks to SIGN in many ways for being the real reason why this is happening! This young generation of surgeons is the future I was talking about that will change fracture care in Ethiopia.

I believe, with the help of SIGN, we have started the right way forward, and in few years, we shall see the standard of care for all the traumas changed! To conclude,

I don't have words enough to thank SIGN and those who have been with me to help me walk again and help others with similar injuries!

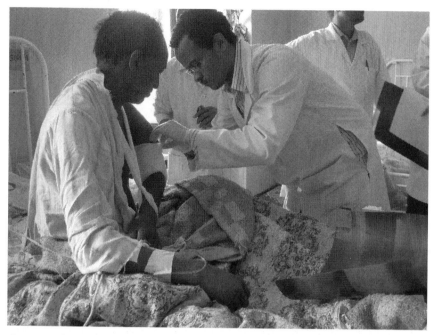

Dr. Sami is a SIGN Patient, a SIGN Surgeon, and a leader. He has organized the first pelvic fracture fellowship in Africa.

After returning from his fellowship in orthopaedic trauma and joint reconstruction in Toronto in 2015, Dr. Sami has established a fellowship to instruct two fellows in the treatment of pelvic fractures. This is the first program in Africa to teach treatment of pelvic fractures. Dr. Sami has offered Dr. Mapuor Mading, from South Sudan, a three-month fellowship in pelvic and acetabular surgery. Dr. Mapuor will then return to his home country, where he will be the only surgeon who can care for these complex fractures.

The rewards of working with the SIGN Family are shown in the faces and the words of patients and surgeons in this chapter. Writing this book has brought back many memories. I rarely look back because the present and future hold many challenges and opportunities to help those who depend on others when injured.

Just as each injury is different, each patient and surgeon is different. Overriding this is the common spark—an equal spark of humanity in us all.

Chapter 12

The Contemplative SIGN Traveler

"When you travel, you don't go to find things, you go to find yourself." —Unknown author

Sharing your skills, experience, and resources brings a new dimension to travel. Volunteering as a medical professional with SIGN will challenge you, provide personal satisfaction from teaching something useful, inspire you with the talent and enthusiasm of SIGN Surgeons who work under difficult conditions, facilitate meaningful friendships with those surgeons, and allow you to see and experience some of the world's most remarkable places.

When you visit a SIGN Program, you and the host surgeons will learn about each other. Some volunteer surgeons teach by seeing patients on the ward, while others like to teach in surgery. Some do both. We all have different gifts to share. We also have different biases. These biases are probably more evident to others than to ourselves. And often, as a volunteer, you will confront your biases when you hear questions like, "Why do you do it that way back home?" The consequences of realizing our own personal biases by having them challenged can lead to wonderful learning experiences. "Why can't a SIGN Tibial Nail be used in the femur?" and "Why can't a SIGN

Nail be used to treat hip fractures?" for example, were questions that challenged me and led to many positive changes.

The volunteer experience can be daunting. You are confronted by a lack of equipment and supplies that we take for granted at home. Many times the patient does not come to the hospital for more than three weeks after an injury. Patients are often treated initially by "bonesetters" who promise to heal the fracture without surgery. This delays and often complicates treatment. Many patients are transferred from hospitals that only have traction. These patients often request their transfer after they learn about the benefits of treatment by a surgeon who uses SIGN Implants.

Over time you will fit into the routine of the host surgeons because you both quickly learn what to expect regarding knowledge and skills. Hopefully, you will have studied the problems surgeons face in developing countries. These fracture problems can be different from those in the United States—including open fractures that have become infected due to a delay in treatment and high-energy fractures caused by road traffic accidents and violence.

Most volunteers relish the experience of assisting in surgery for a patient solely for the benefit of the patient. Although the lack of some supplies can be frustrating, the absence of electronic medical records, insurance forms, and requests for authorization is delightful. As you develop your tactile skills, the surgery will flow because you won't have to stop and look at a screen of instant imaging. You can focus on the procedure. This flow in surgery is pure joy! We become connected with our surgical team and patient, as we all have a common goal. You will welcome the challenge, learn new skills, and you will be inspired. Meeting these challenges creates a surge of creativity and enthusiasm for treating patients who have no other hope.

With proper planning and communication, host surgeons will find patients that have problems in which you are interested or in which you have expertise in solving. We must remember we are there to fill their needs and not our own, but the host surgeons will accommodate your wishes as much as possible. Patients for whom you have done their surgery or assisted with their surgery may return for follow-up care. I remember three Maasai people over age 65 with fractured femurs. They had had these fractures for four years, three years, and two years, respectively. They hadn't sought medical help because they could not afford it. They had expected to have to crawl for the rest of their lives. But when they came for follow-up care, they walked and smiled radiantly.

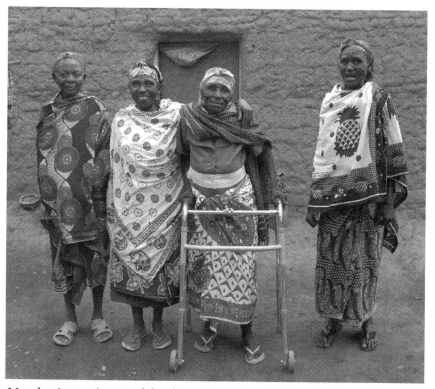

Martha (center), one of the three Maasai patients, is welcomed home by her daughter and neighbors.

You may operate long hours because patients come to the hospital at all times of the day and night. I was at a conference in Tanzania when a woman presented with a severely fractured femur around seven o'clock in the evening. She had been assaulted by her husband. At the same time, there was a banquet scheduled for all members of the conference. There was a delay in preparing the patient for surgery, and we didn't get started until eight o'clock that night. The staff provided the best care they had available. I remember thinking that operating on this poor woman was a privilege far greater than attending a banquet.

If you visit SIGN Programs in developing parts of the world, you will learn to appreciate regional differences that make the surgeons and patients distinct. Mongolian surgeons, for example, are very strong. Their fingers are twice the size of mine and they use them skillfully. They often use their brute strength to reduce fractures that would normally require a mechanical distractor. Mongolian bone is very hard and dense, a consequence, perhaps, of their diets rich in milk and protein, and a nomadic life spent walking and trekking. Vietnamese people, in contrast, have softer long bones while their surgeons have large intrinsic muscles in their hands and demonstrate excellent fine motor control. These differences among people are interesting, but I have found that the similarities among the patients and surgeons from place to place are far more gratifying. Whether you are in Ulaanbaatar or Ho Chi Minh City, you will find dedicated surgeons and grateful patients.

During your stay, you will see patients on the floor between beds, in the hallways, and beds with two patients, either hoping for their time in surgery or recovering from surgery. Many of the fractures treated are more severe than fractures you may be accustomed to treating. You will develop great respect for SIGN Surgeons who accept all patients regardless of complexity of the problem or ability to pay.

There has always been a role for volunteers at SIGN. As SIGN continues to grow, so will our need for volunteers who want to travel abroad and work with SIGN Surgeons. We have, in the past, welcomed volunteers who are not orthopaedic surgeons. I hope that in the future we can find opportunities for professionals who have skills in rehabilitative medicine, operating room administration, physical therapy, and data management as well as specialists in orthopaedics, spine, trauma, tumor, hand, foot and ankle, and neurosurgery.

The volunteer experience with SIGN Fracture Care International is unique. It can last as long as a few days or extend to a few years. It can happen in Asia, Africa, or the Middle East—virtually anywhere in the developing world. It can be one of the most rewarding experiences of your life because it provides a chance to relieve suffering and, often, an enjoyable path to travel and "go find yourself."

Chapter 13

The Journey Continues

Imagine you're running on a treadmill that cannot be stopped and the speed keeps increasing. This describes the journey of SIGN because the number of poor patients injured by trauma, especially road traffic accidents, continues to accelerate. The SIGN Model of education plus donation of appropriate implants is working well, but we must evaluate our model to provide more efficient surgery for increasing numbers of patients.

Surgery is a complex procedure, and the process of healing is very complex. We must avoid the illusion that we know the best way to treat fractures. The history of orthopaedic treatment and pro-gressive changes in surgical implants reminds me that we stand on the shoulders of giants as we innovate new ideas. In addition, SIGN Surgeons continually learn from each other as we review cases on the SIGN Database and discuss new ideas at conferences.

Education is dependent upon communication of ideas as we apply ideas from basic science and innovate uses of implants to promote healing. The annual SIGN Conference in Richland, WA, provides an opportunity for the surgeons in developing countries to present their ideas in their studies of multiple patients to validate these ideas. Regional conferences in developing countries are becoming more numerous and beneficial for better treatment of patients.

The SIGN Database is our main connecting medium because each surgery must be reported on the SIGN Database to receive donated replacement implants. As we analyze large numbers of patients, we note patterns and continue to study them. I review the database every day that I am in the United States. The comment section of the database facilitates exchanges of ideas. I feel thankful and humble that SIGN is playing a big role in treating difficult fractures in developing countries. My humility increases when I read the follow-up reports showing excellent results from treating difficult fractures.

The SIGN IT Department is continually revising our database to improve communication among the SIGN Family. We are realizing that people in developing countries are more likely to use phones than computers to communicate, and we are adapting to this.

SIGN Staff have developed a platform where pelvic fracture x-rays can be sent for evaluation by mentors. The mentor can draw the proposed position of plate stabilization on preoperative x-rays and the SIGN Surgeon can then make a treatment plan. The postoperative x-rays showing the plates holding the fractures in place are then sent to the platform. This is a work in progress, but we are very pleased with our entry into treating pelvic fractures.

Pelvic fractures are very disabling if not treated properly and in a timely basis. The first pelvic fracture fellowship program in Africa is being developed by Dr. Sami Hailu in Ethiopia. Dr. Sami took a one-year fellowship in pelvic fracture and implant surgery in Toronto, Canada, and will be sharing what he learned with other surgeons in East Africa. The C-arm machines in his hospital often do not work, so he does pelvic fracture surgery without instant x-ray imaging. Acumed donated 10 sets of pelvic fracture instruments for SIGN Surgeons to use. SIGN Education is expanding in pelvic fracture surgery as well as SIGN Surgery.

The second part of our model is donation of appropriate implants and instruments. SIGN Staff continues to collaborate with surgeons to learn new ways to use our present implants. We innovate instruments and implants to provide better stabilization of fractures. Observations on the database and suggestions from SIGN Surgeons stimulate these innovations. We all look at fractures with new eyes and develop a fresh approach to fracture treatment. SIGN Surgeons are not bound by conventional wisdom.

We are addressing the biological healing of fractures by using stem cells in cortical bone to accelerate fracture healing. SIGN Engineers, with help from Randy Huebner, developed a bone graft system that includes intramedullary reamers, a reamer flute scraper, and a bone mill to utilize the patient's own bone healing material. We released a new reamer design in 2016 that allows the surgeon to collect more bone marrow and cortical bone shavings containing stem cell particles while preparing the patient's bone canal for SIGN Nail insertion. The Bone Mill is a new device that grinds larger bone fragments that contain stem cells into smaller chips, which can be grafted into the fracture site. Studies indicate that cortical bone contains stem cells and imparting mechanical energy to shave or grind the bone into small particles stimulates the stem cells and promotes fracture healing.

Open fractures are more numerous in developing countries due to the high-energy trauma like road traffic accidents. Established protocol is to provide early antibiotic administration and remove debris and dead tissue from the opening in the skin before stabilizing the fracture. Often this procedure is repeated many times. The question is whether surgical treatment can remove all the bacteria from the wound. I doubt it. The timing of wound closure and placement of the stabilizing implants is being studied by orthopaedic surgeons throughout the world. Bacteria are becoming resistant to antibiotics, so we must look at different protocols which can be applied in our SIGN Programs in developing countries. The first step is to look at timing of soft-tissue closure and placement of the SIGN Nail, and then study other possibilities for better results. We are open to different treatments such as honey and silver to treat the contamination, and then evaluate critically the type of stabilization implants used.

The increasing numbers of fracture patients in developing countries must be addressed. I thought we needed to build new trauma centers based on the model in the United States to meet these increasing numbers of fracture patients. In recent trips I learned that SIGN Surgeons are addressing this by gradual changes in protocol. The number of operating rooms and surgical personnel available must be considered as we seek to increase access to trauma care in developing countries.

The number of orthopaedic surgeons is increasing as new residency programs are formed and residency programs accept more residents. Ethiopia is a prime example of addressing this problem. In 2011 they had 43 orthopaedic surgeons for 100 million people. In 2017 there are 77 orthopaedic residents in training at Black Lion Hospital and 26 residents at St. Paul Hospital, both in Addis Ababa. These newly trained orthopaedic surgeons will request SIGN Implants when they leave to work in other hospitals throughout Ethiopia.

St. Paul Hospital has a policy now of treating patients with fractures on the day they enter the hospital. The patients are discharged the next day or the day after, depending on when they are stable walking on crutches. This helps increase the number of patients that can be treated. Fractures heal faster with earlier surgery. We are also evaluating the treatment of open fractures and timing of external fixation versus placement of a SIGN Nail. Other hospitals are watching these developments and implementing similar protocols.

If there are no operating rooms available in the evening and night and no infrastructure to build new operating rooms, new facilities must be considered. These new facilities will enable surgeons to treat fractures soon after arrival at the hospital. Patients will be discharged the following day or once they are stable on crutches. More complex fractures can be treated with better results. These new facilities will become training centers. Patients will tell others, who will know where to go immediately after injury rather than delay treatment. Treatment is often delayed now due to financial concerns and by bone setters.

The SIGN Family looks backward to learn more and looks forward to improve and extend our vision of creating equality of fracture care throughout the world. We have accomplished a great deal, treating 200,000 patients and counting, but we will not be satisfied until every patient in the world has access to the care needed to heal their injuries.

Please join us on this journey of healing.

Lord, grant that I may always desire more than I can accomplish —A prayer of Michelangelo

★ ★ ★ ★ ★

Dr. Zirkle would like to hear from you. Please send your ideas, questions, or comments to **wewalktheworld@signfracturecare.org**

★ ★ ★ ★ ★

At Dr. Zirkle's request, all proceeds from this book will be donated to SIGN Fracture Care International.

Appendix

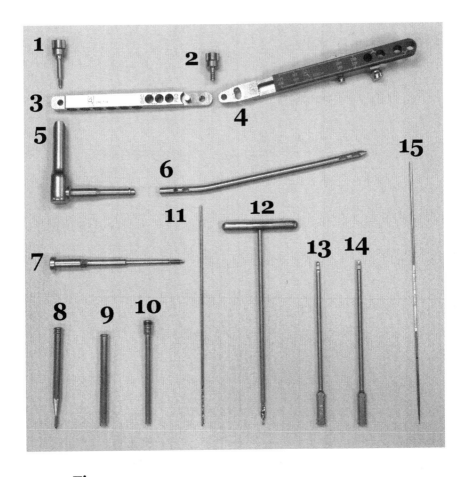

Figure 1

Basic SIGN Instruments

1   Shoulder Cap Screw

2   Adjustment Screw

3	Target Arm—Proximal Section
4	Target Arm—Distal Extension and Center Section
5	L Handle
6	SIGN Nail
7	Locking Bolt—fits through L handle and attaches nail to target arm
8	Alignment Pin
9	Cannula-fits into round holes of distal target arm to guide and secure various drills, drill guides, step drill, and slot finders
10	Drill Guide
11	Small Drill Bit—3.5 mm
12	Step Drill—enlarges the 3.5 drill hole to insert the slot finders and engage larger diameter threads on the head of the screw
13	Solid Slot Finder
14	Cannulated Slot Finder
15	Depth gauge—to determine interlocking screw length

* * * * *

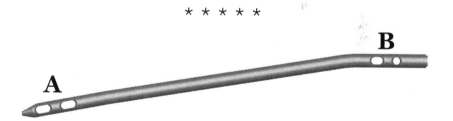

Figure 2

The SIGN Nail is made of solid 316 L surgical-grade stainless steel. It has two slots at the distal end (A) and a round hole, a slot, and a 9° bend (B) at the proximal end. Nail diameters range from 8-12 mm (5/16"-1/2") in 1 mm increments, with lengths from 200-420 mm (9.6"-17") in 20 mm increments.

Figure 3

The 316 L stainless steel SIGN L Interlocking Screw is self-tapping with a recessed hexagonal socket. It comes in lengths from 25-75 mm (1-3"). The central shaft is non-threaded, giving the screw added strength.

* * * * *

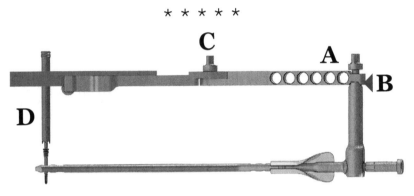

Figure 4

The proximal target arm is attached to the assembled L handle with the shoulder cap screw (A). The dual tapered design of this junction (B) is precise, insuring the accurate targeting of the distal slots with the target arm.

The distal target arm is attached to the proximal target arm with an adjustment screw (C). The distal extension and center section have a sliding feature allowing the target arm to be lengthened and shortened for use with various lengths of SIGN Nails. The alignment pin (D) passes through a distal targeting hole of the target arm and engages the most distal slot in the nail to make angular adjustments as necessary and confirm alignment.

Confirmation of accurate alignment before the nail is placed in the bone reassures the surgeon that all the parts of the nail and targeting system line up. At this point the target arm is disassembled from the L handle, and the nail is introduced into the intramedullary canal of the bone using a pushing/twisting motion on the L handle or gently tapping on the head of the locking bolt with a mallet until the nail is seated.

★ ★ ★ ★ ★

Procedure for Distal Targeting

The target arm is reassembled onto the L handle. The cannula is inserted through the appropriate distal targeting hole in the target arm and placed on the bone surface. The cannula is held steady by an assistant during drilling.

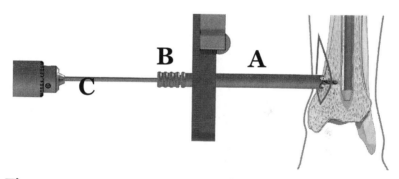

Figure 5
Using the cannula (A) and the small drill guide (B) as a guide the 3.5mm drill bit (C) is drilled through the near bone cortex only.

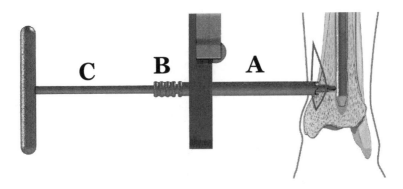

Figure 6

Keeping the cannula (A) in place, the small drill guide is replaced by the large drill guide (B). The 3.5mm drill hole is enlarged with a step drill (C). When the flattened tip of the step drill engages the nail's slot, it will cease moving.

* * * * *

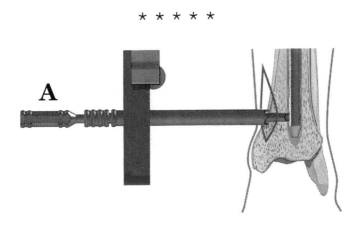

Figure 7

The oval end of the solid slot finder (A) is inserted through the large drill guide and bone until it engages the nail's slot. When the slot finder is properly seated in the slot, it will only rotate through a jog of 10-15°. This is the "SIGN Feel."

The cannulated slot finder replaces the solid slot finder.

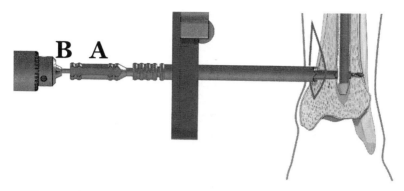

Figure 8

With the cannulated slot finder (A) in the nail's slot, the 3.5mm drill (B) drills the far bone cortex. A depth gauge measures the screw size.

* * * * *

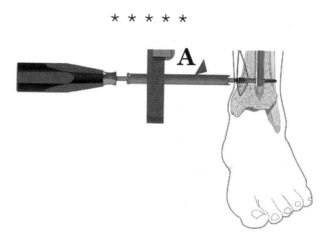

Figure 9

The SIGN Interlocking Screw (A) is inserted through the cannula to engage both bone cortices and the nail.

Inability of the surgeon to pull or twist the nail out from the intramedullary canal confirms that the nail is locked to the bone. The second distal locking screw and the two proximal locking screws are placed in like manner. The target arm, locking bolt, and L handle are removed and the incisions closed.

Glossary

Acetabular—relating to the acetabulum, the cavity at the base of the hip bone where the ball of the femur fits

Anterior—situated near or toward the head or top of a bone

Arthroplasty—the surgical reconstruction or replacement of a joint

Arthroscope—an instrument through which the interior of a joint may be inspected or operated on

Bonesetter—traditional healer with skill in manipulation, bandaging of extremity injuries, but without access to x-rays or modern medical facilities

C-arm—an x-ray machine and monitor that shows real-time x-ray pictures, also called fluoroscope or image intensifier

Cortex—the hard outer wall of a bone

Didactic—intended for instruction

Distal—away from the center, or away from the point of reference. In the SIGN Nail, the distal end is the furthest from the end that couples with the inserting instruments

Distractor—device that pulls bone fragments apart so that a surgeon can reset them in proper alignment for healing

Femur—bone of the upper leg

Humerus—bone of the upper arm

Intramedullary—within the marrow cavity of a bone. An intramedullary (IM) nail is inserted into the bone cavity to hold two ends of a fractured long bone in position, so it can heal

Malalignment—Incorrect or imperfect alignment of bones, often leading to deformity or reduced function of the limb

Medullary canal—the marrow cavity of a bone

Necrotic—cell or tissues that have died due to inadequate blood supply, bacterial infection, traumatic injury, or hyperthermia

Olecranon—the bony prominence of the elbow

Osteotomy—a surgical operation in which a bone is divided or a piece of bone is excised (as to correct a deformity)

Patella—a thick flat triangular movable bone that forms the anterior point of the knee and protects the front of the joint, also known as the kneecap

Pedicle—a short, stem-like projection located on the backside of a vertebral body in the spine

Perfusion—the passage of fluid through the circulatory system or lymphatic system to an organ or a tissue, usually referring to the delivery of blood to a capillary bed in tissue

Physeal Plate—the region in a long bone between the epiphysis and diaphysis where growth in length occurs, also known as the growth plate

Posterior—near or toward the back of the body

Proximal—near to or close. In the SIGN Nail, the end that is coupled with the insertion instruments

Reamer—a rotating tool with cutting edges used to enlarge or shape a hole, used to enlarge the intramedullary canal before inserting a nail

Retrocalcaneal fusion—the surgical procedure of inserting a SIGN Nail through the bottom of a foot, through the ankle joint, and into the tibia. This is used to fuse the ankle joint.

Retrograde—the retrograde approach to the femur is from the end of the bone near the knee, rather than the antegrade approach from the hip

Schanz Pins—small metal pins used to connect the external fixation device to the bone

Sensate—capable of perceiving sensory stimuli

Traction (orthopaedic)—a way of treating broken bones in which a device gently pulls the bones back into place

Tibia—the shin bone

Trochanter—a rough prominence at the upper part of the femur, serving for the attachment of muscles

Editors' Note:

Some quotes and passages written by SIGN Surgeons in **We Walk the World** *have been slightly altered for grammar and to match the style of the book, or to protect the identity of individuals in dangerous areas. Our goal is to provide clarity for the reader while maintaining the intent and voice of the original author.*

About the Author

Lewis G. Zirkle, MD, is a board certified orthopaedic surgeon who maintained a thriving private practice for more than 40 years in Richland, WA. He graduated from Davidson College and Duke University Medical Center. After one year in the orthopaedic residency program at Duke University Medical Center, he was drafted into the US Army and sent to Vietnam. He continued his training in the Army. Dr. Zirkle has traveled extensively in developing countries to teach orthopaedic surgery since 1970. In 1999, he founded SIGN Fracture Care International (SIGN), where orthopaedic implants and instruments are designed, manufactured, and donated to surgeons in developing countries to be used in austere operating theaters.

Since SIGN was founded, Dr. Zirkle has spent increasing amounts of time engaged in development of new surgical implants that can be used in developing countries, developing curriculum applicable to the surgeons, and traveling to teach surgery and modern orthopaedic care. He is known throughout the orthopaedic community as the main catalyst for enabling orthopaedic surgeons in developing countries to provide immediate and effective surgical care to their patients. Thousands of people can attribute their mobility to his dedication.

Dr. Zirkle is a man of incredible energy, creativity, and courage. He has traveled to areas of conflict such as Pakistan, Afghanistan, and Iraq to provide equipment and training, and has answered to calls for help during disasters, including Haiti and Nepal. He has won many awards for his commitment, including the AAOS Humanitarian award in 2007 and the Allama Sayed Jamaluddin Medal from Afghanistan in 2015.

He lives and works in Richland, Washington, with his wife Dr. Sara Zirkle and their granddog Rex.

Made in the USA
Lexington, KY
25 September 2017